Traditional Chinese Medicine

Tribute to Professor Rod Gerber

Why thunder strikes on a clear day?
Why a noble person should be taken away?
The news of his death stabbed me, and I cried like an unceasing torrent.

I pause for a moment. Memories of him and the blessings I received flooding in: the unfailing encouraging words, the constant positive remarks, and the humanistic way, mingled with his sense of humour.

Professor Rod Gerber was my mentor, my teacher, my co-researcher, and spiritual leader, from whom I learnt in so many ways.

Reflections of life and death reminded me of the ancient sayings, such as Zeus, in Greek myths, about the charm of mortality:

We miss the poignancy of the transience, the sweet sadness of grasping for something we know we cannot hold.

And as Lao Tzu, the ancient Chinese philosopher, said about the unity of humans and nature (Professor Rod Gerber was receptive of Tao), and death was as much a part of nature as life, 'exiting life, we enter death' (*Tao Te Ching*, chapter 50).

Though he is gone, his spirit lives on, and in my heart.

Traditional Chinese Medicine

The Human Dimension

Big Leung PhD

中醫藥
以人為本

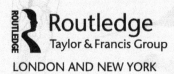

Routledge
Taylor & Francis Group

LONDON AND NEW YORK

First published 2008 by Goshawk Publishing

Published in 2016
by Routledge
2 Park Square, Milton Park, Abingdon, Oxon OX14 4RN
711 Third Avenue, New York, NY, 10017, USA

Routledge is an imprint of the Taylor & Francis Group, an informa business

National Library of Australia Cataloguing-in-Publication data
Leung, Big, 1958– .
Traditional chinese medicine: the human dimension.

Bibliography.
Includes index.
ISBN 978 0 9775742 2 3 (pbk.).

1. Medicine, Chinese. 2. China – Social life and customs.
3. China – Civilization. I. Title.

610.951

ISBN 13: 9780977574223 (pbk)

Foreword

项 序

中华文化上下五千年，源远流长；岐黄医学洋洋两千载，博大精深。中医药学乃中国传统文化之艳丽瑰宝、璀灿明珠，其以中国古代丰富的医疗实践经验的积累为基础，吸取并运用了中国古代的哲学学说，如精气学说、阴阳学说、五行学说等，从而使之具有深厚的中华文化底蕴。可见，中医药学与中国文化密切相关，其不仅为中华民族的繁衍昌盛作出了杰出贡献，而且为世界上越来越多的国家和地区民众乃至政府所欢迎。WHO也十分重视和支持中医药的发展，中医药学已经成为世界医学之林中的一朵绚丽奇葩，为保障全人类的健康发挥了重要作用。

Big Leung女士熟悉中华文化，热爱中医药事业，深知学习中华文化，推广应用中医药学对促进人类健康水平提高的意义。她在广泛收集资料，深入进行研究的基础上，历时×年编写成此书。本书的出版发行，定能让世界上更多的人通过阅读本书了解中华文化，学习和应用中医药的基本知识，以指导养生保健和对疾病的防治，从而为增进人类健康作出贡献。乐此善举，欣然为序。

澳门科技大学中医药学院 项 平　　二〇〇七年九月于澳门

Chinese culture has a long history of over five thousand years, whereas the profound knowledge of Chinese medicine in China has accumulated for over two thousand years. Within the realm of Chinese culture, Chinese medicine is a precious gem, like a glittering pearl, embedded in a wealth of practical experience and ancient Chinese philosophies: the concepts of Qi, Yin–Yang, Five Elements, all of which are deep-rooted in the Chinese cultural heritage. They reflect the close correspondence of Traditional Chinese Medicine and Chinese culture.

Traditional Chinese Medicine is one of China's major contributions to the world, and is sought after by many countries, various localities and governments around the world. World Health Organisation (WHO) also recognises and supports the development of Traditional Chinese Medicine. Traditional Chinese Medicine has become a major player on the world stage for its pivotal role in safeguarding world health.

Big Leung possesses good knowledge of Chinese culture, with a commitment toward employing Traditional Chinese Medicine as a method for the advancement of health standard. She conducted extensive research, employing diverse sources of reference materials and techniques; her endeavour in writing this book was done through many years of hard work. The publication of this book will contribute to the understanding of Chinese culture, the fundamental knowledge of Traditional Chinese Medicine for health preservation and disease prevention. Based on her noble pursuit of excellence in the humanities, I am honoured to write this Foreword.

Professor Xiang Ping (项 平), former President of Nanjing University of Traditional Chinese Medicine, Dean, Faculty of Chinese Medicine, Macau University of Science and Technology, Macau September, 2007 (translated by the author)

Foreword

Traditional Chinese Medicine is considered alternative medicine in the West, whereas in China it is considered to be an integral part of the health care system. The phrase TCM was coined by the People's Republic of China to promote Chinese medicine in the wider world. Processes of the human body are, in TCM theory, interrelated and in constant interaction with the environment. The TCM practitioner sees signs of disharmony which are understood and treated, and further illness and disease prevented. TCM is commonly used to treat cravings and withdrawal symptoms of smokers and other addicts, the side effects of chemotherapy and many chronic conditions. Big Leung discusses the philosophical frameworks of TCM theory, including the Five Elements, Yin–Yang, the Meridian system and others as integral to a consideration of human centredness.

The Human Dimension is seen in terms of Humanism, a broad category of ethical philosophies that affirm the dignity and worth of all people. Humanism sees as intrinsic a commitment to the search for morality and truth through human means to support the interests of humans. Humanists support the principle of universal morality based on the universality of our human condition and see our human culture and social problems in the wider context.

Chinese culture is central to the author's purpose and she is concerned particularly with the cultural problems faced by the Chinese diaspora. Traditional Chinese medicine is a pivotal strength of many, far from their homeland in time and geography. Big Leung has found that participants in her study often perceived TCM as Chinese culture, and as an important vehicle for realizing idealistic principles that connect with significant Traditional Chinese cultural values, as instanced by human centredness, and she believes the words of Tang Chun I that 'The essence of Chinese culture resides in humanism, the human heart'. Humanism in Confucianism, Mohism and Taoism is explored, as is the concept of Yin and Yang, intrinsic to Chinese understanding of harmony and balance. She applies these principles to youth, adulthood and old age.

TCM links the family and she covers this important area in her chapter on family connectedness before considering the question of identity and conceptions of leadership in TCM. Throughout her writing Big Leung sees the importance of harmony and balance – balance through Yin and Yang, balancing emotions, balance with the environment and the important matter of balance in food, described as the essence of life in Nei Jing. Disease is seen to result from imbalance.

I commend this book to all those who seek a greater understanding of the role of TCM, particularly among the Chinese diaspora.

Congratulations Big. Well done. You have worked hard and I wish you every success with this book.

Dr Gerald Brereton Heyner Lewis, MB BS, MLitt, MRehab C'ling, PhD Acupuncture, MD(MA), DSc(Hon), FFARACS, FANZCA
Formerly Assistant Professor of Anaesthesia, University of Saskatchewan Canada.
Director of the Pain Clinic, Armidale Regional Rural Referral Hospital,
Hunter New England Health Region, New South Wales, Australia

Contents

CHAPTER ONE 連 (Pronounced as *lin*, which means 'connections')

CHAPTER TWO 仁 (Pronounced as *lans*, which means 'benevolence' or 'humanism', and 'two people')

CHAPTER THREE 信 (Pronounced as *xin*, which means 'beliefs' in health and human trust)

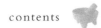

About the author

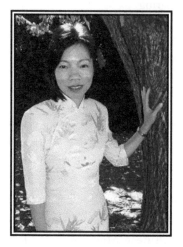

'Big' means the love of nature. Big Leung gained her PhD in the social analysis of Traditional Chinese Medicine at the University of New England, Australia. She has worked in health services (psychiatric and general nursing and administration), studied higher classical Chinese, marketing and management, and has been involved in voluntary social work. Before migrating to Australia, she lived in Macau, Hong Kong, London and Canton. She has travelled widely in Europe, Canada and the United States. Her passion in research resides in social and cultural studies in the fields of health and humanities. Apart from English, she can speak Cantonese, Mandarin and See Yup dialect, and has many friends around the world.

About the cover design

Since ancient times, Chinese people have gathered plants from the mountains for use as medicines. Indeed, participants in studies reported in this book recalled their own parents gathering herbs from the mountains to prepare as Traditional Chinese Medicine for family members, carrying this age-old tradition through into modern times.

The three human figures, young, middle-aged and old, male and female, represent the participants in these studies. The female figure is depicted as a caring mother with a loving healthy image, as is reflected in participants' stories.

THE ARTIST
Michael Chun, the author's brother-in-law, contributed the artwork for the book cover.

CHINESE CHARACTERS
Kee-chi Leung, the author's brother, contributed the calligraphy that appears on the title page.

Preface

To me, Traditional Chinese Medicine means human expressions and connections, imbued with profound Chinese cultural values.

My social interaction with Traditional Chinese Medicine began at home when I was a child. My mother used to say I was born a healthy baby because she had taken ginseng and bird's nest during her pregnancy, and that I grew into a healthy child because she continued to give me Traditional Chinese Medicine. My childhood memories of Traditional Chinese Medicine are of herbal teas and soups, some for keeping the body cool or warm, some for good complexion, and others, shared among family members, for general good health. Where I grew up in Macau and Hong Kong, there were many shops selling a wide variety of Traditional Chinese Medicine remedies and ready-made herbal drinks. Traditional Chinese Medicine was an integral part of life for the Chinese people who lived there.

In undertaking the two research projects reported in this book, my passion was to do something about and for Chinese people. My investigations into Traditional Chinese Medicine were from the perspective of social science — studying the social and cultural meanings of Traditional Chinese Medicine, rather than its effectiveness and use.

In the earlier research project (for my PhD, mainly reported in chapters three to seven), I interviewed Chinese people living in Armidale, Brisbane and Sydney (all in Australia) who had experienced early life in countries such as Mainland China, Taiwan, Hong Kong and other south-east Asian countries, as well as in Papua New Guinea. The human stories associated with these people's experiences of Chinese medicine intrigued me. Subsequently I interviewed Chinese people in Macau and Hong Kong to explore their conceptions of leadership in Traditional Chinese Medicine, under the guidance of Professor Rod Gerber (who is acknowledged as co-author of the study as reported in chapter eight).

During the course of writing this book, I have felt a heavy responsibility to bring out the best core values of Chinese culture, values that can be applied in the modern world. In my heart I deeply believe that the real strength and prosperity of a culture resides not just in material riches but also in its social and philosophical achievements, through which people benefit by being able to experience life in a more harmonious way. My conviction about this human dimension in Traditional Chinese Medicine has been shaped by my personal experiences as well as by the experiences of life that others have shared with me.

My understanding of this humanistic orientation has developed through my involvement in social activities in schools and voluntary work in the community and, in particular, from my classical Chinese studies after I finished high school and my training, in London, as a nurse. I remember well the first lesson in nursing school: to be 'patient-centred'.

My subsequent experiences with people of various nationalities and places have further reinforced my belief in humanism. I visited Canada and the United States of America four months after the September 11 2001 attacks on the Twin Towers in New York. I visited a friend who told me of how the daughter of one of her friends had been a victim of the September 11th tragedy. She had been at her first job, fresh from college and full of hope. I felt deeply for this young woman, her family and her friends.

A few years later, in 2004, I attended a symposium in Melbourne, Australia, which touched on terrorism. Speaker after speaker recounted man's inhumanity toward man – the September 11 attack, the Bali disaster... the untold waste of human lives. I could not control myself and burst into inconsolable tears. There have been more shocking terrorist attacks, such as the London bombing in 2005. The London underground was a familiar place to me and had been one of my favourite modes of transport when I lived there. I wondered why that peaceful landscape should be disturbed.

More recently, I met a group of visiting scholars from Iraq. I learnt about their war-torn country, their hardship, their sense of physical danger and psychological insecurity. There seemed to be no tomorrow for them. I remember the despair and fear revealed in their eyes, the yearning for hope and peace echoing in their voices.

I believe the meanings of medicine and life are intertwined. Most significantly, the practice and experience of Traditional Chinese Medicine stimulates our thinking about how to live in a more humane way. This is the passion I wish to share with you.

I have enjoyed writing this book. Any errors are my sole responsibility. I welcome all constructive comments.

Big Leung PhD
July 2007
Armidale NSW, AUSTRALIA

Acknowledgements

Writing a book is an enriching experience. I remember with sincere thanks the people who have had positive impacts on me during this journey, either by sharing their knowledge or by sustaining my emotional wellbeing, or both.

This book would not have been realised without the data from my PhD research (mainly chapters three to seven) and another research study (chapter eight). I have enjoyed the enthusiasm and unreserved support of the Chinese participants in Armidale, Brisbane and Sydney (all in Australia), Macau and Hong Kong, and Western participants in Brisbane (Australia). Through their stories of their experiences with Traditional Chinese Medicine, I have learnt of medicine and of the depth and breadth of the connection between Traditional Chinese Medicine and people.

I cannot thank enough James Davidson, the Publishing Director of Verdant House, for his insights, trust, support and positive attitude toward my work. I acknowledge the members of the team who contributed to the production of this book. I am grateful to Eve Witney, editor, for her time and energy in strengthening the manuscript. Thanks also go to Karen Enkelaar for the page concept and to Kim Webber for the desktop publishing and cover design.

My sincere gratitude to the following academics/professionals who gave of their time and expertise in reading, commenting on, and in some cases editing sections of this book:

Professor Alan Atkinson, Historian and Australia Research Council Professorial Fellow, School of Classics, History, and Religion, University of New England (Australia), for editing and commenting on the chapter about family connectedness.

Dr Nicholas Bunnin, Philosopher at the Institute for Chinese Studies, University of Oxford (Britain) (referred by Professor Glen Dudbridge), for commenting on the chapter about the human-centred nature of traditional Chinese culture.

Professor Barney Glaser (United States of America), sociologist, publisher and co-founder of grounded theory methodology, who commented on an early draft of the section about the social meanings of Traditional Chinese Medicine.

Professor Rod Gerber, Senior Academic Advisor, Qantm College, Brisbane (Australia) and Director of Research and Publication at SAE International Graduate College, for reading the chapter about balance and harmony.

Professor Lynn Meek, Educational Management, Head of the School of Professional Development and Leadership Studies, University of New England (Australia), for reading the chapter about leadership in Traditional Chinese Medicine.

Associate Professor Michael Sharkey, Poet, School of English, Communication, and Theatre, University of New England (Australia), for reading an early draft of the chapter about the human-centred nature of traditional Chinese culture.

Sam Wong AM, Principal Government Pharmacist, TGA (Australia), who also provided helpful feedback, from a lay perspective, on an early draft of the section about the social meanings of Traditional Chinese Medicine.

My gratitude goes to Professor Rod Gerber, who introduced me to various qualitative methods. I treasure his encouragement, positive thinking and, above all, contributions to my intellectual activity.

I am blessed by the care of my brothers, Calvin and Kee-chi, and sisters, Emily and Cynthia, and their lovely families. In particular, I thank Emily and Calvin for their unconditional support over the years. I am grateful to Michael, my brother-in-law, for undertaking to provide the painting for the book cover, and to my brother, Kee-chi, for writing the book title in Chinese calligraphy (which appears on the title page).

Friends are an important part of my life, and all my friends around the world in some way help me to see life in a more colourful way. I appreciate modern technology, such as email, mobile phones and telephones, which shortens the distance between us. I would like to express a note of respect to all my elderly friends (70 to 100 years of age), in particular the Aboriginal elders and Europeans friends whom I visit as a volunteer in Armidale (Australia). Through them I have felt the comfort of having parents and grandparents.

Through my two sons, Andrew and Tannoy, I have a different experience of life – the joy and pain of being a mother. I express a special note of pride to Tannoy, who was there, providing inspiring background music while I wrote this book, and offering computer support whenever I needed it.

Finally, my deepest respect to my loving father and mother, Hung Leung and Chui-yuet Woo, my grandfather and grandmother, See-ting Leung and Yuk-mui Lee, and my adopted British grandmother, Hilda E. Bake (of London), whose caring spirits are always with me.

I treasure the experiences, the social interactions, and the knowledge that I have gained through the journey of writing this book. I will continue to develop my understanding of health, medicine and humans.

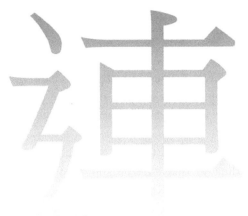

chapter one

Traditional Chinese Medicine: The Connections

(Pronounced as *lin*, which means 'connections')

Traditional Chinese Medicine is a human phenomenon, connecting people in the world.

Ancient Chinese people developed the wisdom of Traditional Chinese Medicine through their timeless efforts in coping with health and illness. Traditional Chinese Medicine has become a system of healing and a Chinese health discipline grounded in ancient philosophical texts. Early Chinese medical thought has been greatly influenced by Tao and *yin* and *yang* theory, which emphasise harmony with nature and co-operation, and that all relationships are complementary. An excess or a deficiency in either *yin* or *yang* is thought to be a prelude to illness.

Practitioners and users of Traditional Chinese Medicine characteristically focus on the whole person, the close correspondence between the individual and nature, and the core principles of balance and harmony which contribute to health and wellbeing. The main effect of disease, according to tradition, is the blockage of *qi*, the vital life force, which permeates our bodies, as well as the universe.

The influence of Traditional Chinese Medicine is widespread throughout the world. According to one estimate, up to one quarter of the world's population, including Chinese, Korean and Japanese people, are thought to be using Traditional Chinese Medicine (Jones & Vincent 1998). The significance of Traditional Chinese Medicine is revealed in its connectedness with Chinese heritage and identity, and as a continuous cultural achievement from China (Leung 2004). Traditional Chinese Medicine plays a significant role as a preference in the delivery of health care among Chinese people both within China and throughout the Chinese diaspora.

To provide a background for understanding the participants' perceptions of Traditional Chinese Medicine presented later in this book, it will be helpful to have an understanding of the historical influences of Western medicine in China and how policy impinges on the concurrent use of these two health systems in China. Further to this, the use of Traditional Chinese Medicine reveals an attachment to traditional Chinese culture by Chinese people throughout the Chinese diaspora and in former European colonies. The extent of Traditional Chinese Medicine use in Australia and in Hong Kong and Macau is also provides perspective for this discussion.

Western Medicine in China

'Western medicine', as a body of theory and practice, started to be consolidated in Western Europe during the fifteenth and sixteenth centuries, incorporating ideas and practices developed by and diffused from various cultures (Ho & Lisowski 1993). Western medicine was introduced to China through the influence of missionaries, the Chinese government, and Chinese individuals interested in learning Western medicine (Andrews 1996).

When the Jesuits brought Western medicine to China in the sixteenth and seventeenth centuries, it was seen as a curiosity; the medical teachings were preserved in a library (Ho & Lisowski 1993). Western medicine was not appreciated at first because of the vast differences between the two medical models in terms of theory and practices. At first, Western medicine was mainly used by low status and poor people who could not afford local doctors, as reported by a missionary:

While the wealthier people do call native doctors, and will continue to do so to some extent, the great class of poorer people, whose conditions of life render them more liable to disease, and who would or could not go to the native doctors, are glad to put themselves under our care.

(Andrews 1996)

Western medicine was introduced through the efforts of some notable people: Dr Alexander Pearson, who introduced vaccination to China (1805); Benjamin Hobson (1816 to 1873), who was believed to have introduced Western medicine into China through his works *Outline of Western Medicine, New Anatomy of the Human Body, New Discourse on Internal Medicine,* and *Simple Discourse on Gynaecology and Paediatrics;* Dr Parker (1834), who introduced chloroform in surgery; John Fryer (1839 to 1928), who translated a great number of the Western medical texts into Chinese (Ho & Lisowski 1993), and the medical missionary John Kerr, who went to Canton in 1854 and ran the Boji Hospital. He worked there for forty-seven years, treating more than one million patients and training medical students (Wikipedia Encyclopedia 2007).

It was during the second half of the nineteenth century that Western medicine underwent a period of further development. Some Western doctors and medical missionaries were successful in coping with infectious diseases by means of vaccination and improved standards of hygiene and public health, establishing the reputation of Western medicine (Porkert & Ullmann 1982).

Western medicine was in a favourable position in China at the turn of the twentieth century for two reasons: firstly, the Chinese government provided support for medical science and a public health program was established; and secondly, scientific methods promised an optimistic outlook (Unschuld 1985).

Dr Sun Yat-sen, the 'Father of Modern China' in Taiwan and China and founder of the Republic of China in 1912, graduated from the Hong Kong College of Medicine for Chinese and received training as a Western medical practitioner at Boji Hospital. He recognised the importance of science in the Republic's Constitution and asserted that: 'What we need to learn from Europe is science, not political philosophy' (in Creel 1975:243). Under the Nationalist regime, Western medicine was favoured. An unsuccessful attempt was made to abolish Traditional Chinese Medicine in the year 1929. The 'unscientific' nature of Traditional Chinese Medicine was one of the reasons it was marginalised at that time. Various institutions were set up for the purpose of incorporating science into Traditional Chinese Medicine, such as the Research

Society for the Improvement of Chinese Medicine, established in 1919, and the Institution for National Medicine, established in 1931 (Penny 1993).

Having Traditional Chinese Medicine working alongside Western medicine became a major health policy in Communist China. During the civil war in the 1930s, Mao Zedong, Chairperson of Communist China, required all medical workers 'to serve the people' (Porkert & Ullmann 1982:260). Driven by necessity, it became obvious that more than one type of health care was needed to serve the massive population:

> In the countryside, where trained physicians were in desperately short supply, the old-style doctors were used on a large scale, but they were almost entirely excluded from the large urban hospitals and government medical institutions.
>
> (Penny 1993:176)

In 1958 Mao Zedong delivered this famous dictum: 'Chinese medicine is a great treasure house! We must make all efforts to uncover it and raise its standards'. In the same year, the Central Committee of the Chinese Communist Party endorsed the co-existence of Western medicine and Traditional Chinese Medicine, stating that they 'should serve side by side' (Porkert & Ullmann 1982:260). In 1982, the Constitution was redrafted to include 'developing modern medicine and traditional medicine of our country', a policy that placed Western medicine and Traditional Chinese Medicine on an equal footing (Shi 1995:9.2).

In recent years the popularity of Western medicine has risen among the younger Chinese generation. In modern China the two medical models not only co-exist, but co-operate to serve the Chinese people (Liu 2006). Three types of medical science are available: Traditional Chinese Medicine, Western medicine, and 'integrated medicine', offering flexibility in health care.

Traditional Chinese Medicine in Australia

Traditional Chinese Medicine is categorised under complementary therapies by the Australian Bureau of Statistics (2001). In 2003 in Australia, an estimated $2.3 billion was spent on complementary alternative medicine (Adams, Sibbritt, Easthope & Young 2003). This figure is more than double the estimate for the year 2000 of $1 billion and, according to research conducted by Australian Consumer Associations about the same time (Choice 2001:1), more than half of the population had used complementary alternative medicine.

Around two-thirds of the amount spent on complementary alternative medicine in Australia is for Traditional Chinese Medicine, according to the *Xinhua News* (19 April 2001). The report on a 1996 stage one research project into Traditional Chinese Medicine practice, commissioned by the Victoria Ministerial Advisory Committee (1998), revealed there are around 2.8 million Traditional Chinese Medicine consultations yearly Australia-wide, which amounts to an annual turnover of $84 million in this sector of Australia's health economy.

As categorised by the Australian Bureau of Statistics, Traditional Chinese Medicine encompasses diverse modalities such as acupuncture, Chinese herbal therapy, massage therapy, dietary therapy, scraping, moxibustion, and exercise therapy such as Qi Gong and Tai Chi. A Traditional Chinese Medicine practitioner is defined under Complementary Health Therapists by the Australian Bureau of Statistics (2006) as:

[One who] treats imbalances of energy flows through the body by assessing the whole person and using techniques and methods such as acupuncture, Chinese herbal medicine, massage, diet, exercise and breathing therapy. Registration or licensing may be required.

In Australia Traditional Chinese Medicine is used, alone or to complement Western medicine, for treating and preventing disease, especially chronic diseases such as cancer, allergies, heart disease and AIDS.

Traditional Chinese Medicine in Hong Kong and Macau

In Hong Kong (a British colony before 1997), a statistics report in the year 2000 indicated there were 1 050 600 persons using Traditional Chinese Medicine, representing 15.5 per cent of the population (C&SD 2000). The number of consultations for Traditional Chinese Medicine was 322 000, accounting for 22.7 per cent of the 1.43 million doctor consultations. Traditional Chinese Medicine was mainly used for regulating the body (63.3 per cent). The majority of users were women between 35 and 54 years of age.

Macau was under Portuguese administration before 1999. The number of Traditional Chinese Medicine consultations in Macau in 2003 was estimated at 597 407, including 63.7 per cent for general treatments, 26.4 per cent for bone-setting, 5.5 per cent for acupuncture, and 4.2 per cent for massage (DCEC 2004).

Investigation of Traditional Chinese Medicine in this book

The discourses of Traditional Chinese Medicine are socially and culturally constructed, as are those of Western medicine. They are complex and conceptual, and require referencing to more concrete social and cultural practices grounded in participants' experiences, beliefs, and interactions with others. The intricate meanings of Traditional Chinese Medicine are congruent with the view that medical experiences, as expressed in *Nei Jing*, the first Chinese Medical Classic, are replete with symbols and meanings and are connected to multiple contemporary ideas (Bary & Bloom 1999). As pointed out by Sivin (2003), the strength of Traditional Chinese Medicine involves complex relationships and is best evaluated through its analysis of how functions on many levels, including the body, emotions, natural and social environments, are related.

Understanding social, cultural and historical contexts helps us to uncover the actions and meanings of individuals in the social world, and to see and feel in a more humane way. Cooley (1926:64) spoke of this as the 'sympathetic elements' which make us 'distinctively human'. Exploring the social knowledge of Traditional Chinese Medicine helps us excite our sociological imaginations (Wright 1959:32) in order to see Traditional Chinese Medicine, a familiar and natural experience to some of us, with new significance.

Traditional Chinese Medicine was often perceived as Chinese culture by participants in this book, and as an important vehicle for realising idealistic principles that connect with significant traditional Chinese cultural values. Understanding these philosophical meanings will help us to appreciate the social and human side of participants' connections with Traditional Chinese Medicine, and with traditional Chinese culture as a whole. Therefore, the book will present the core values in Chinese culture, starting with a detailed discussion of human centredness and its philosophical underpinnings, providing the framework for the exploration of Traditional Chinese Medicine in the following chapters. The various meanings ascribed to Traditional Chinese Medicine by Chinese participants in two studies conducted in Australia (chapter three to seven) and Hong Kong and Macau (chapter eight) are presented. Each chapter features a Chinese character, the meaning of which encompasses the key message of that chapter.

Other features provided at the end of this book – the glossary of Chinese terms, supplementary notes on Chinese philosophers and classic literature, and Chinese metaphors and sayings – contain enlightening reading to further enhance the reader's appreciation of Chinese culture.

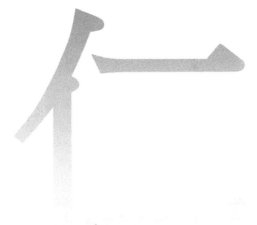

chapter two

The Spirit of Chinese Culture: Its Human Centredness

(Pronounced as *lans*, which means 'benevolence'
or 'humanism', and 'two people')

The essence of Chinese culture resides in humanism, the human heart.

Tang Chun-I 唐君毅 2000

Introduction

The human dimension of Traditional Chinese Medicine uncovers some of the core values of Chinese culture. This chapter serves as the backbone for the following chapters by highlighting how many aspects of traditional Chinese culture are applicable to this modern world. I believe the beauty of Chinese culture is that its essence resides in humanism, in the human heart, a view in line with those of Tang Chun-I (唐君毅), a modern Chinese philosopher, in his monumental work on the spiritual value of Chinese culture (Tang 2000).

Humanism is prominent in Traditional Chinese culture. In the following sections, the relationship of Chinese culture with humans is defined. The historical development of humanism is described, supported by the teachings of Confucianism, Taoism, and Mohism, the main schools of humanistic thinking. The contribution of the underpinning concept of *yin* and *yang* to balance and harmony in life and health is considered. The core values of Chinese culture are explored, embracing the three main human relationships of human and self, human and others, and human and the universe. Finally, the significance of human centredness as applied to this modern world is examined and discussed.

Throughout this chapter, references are drawn primarily from these Chinese classics:

- *I Ching* (易經)
- *Tao Te Ching* (道德經)
- The *Confucian Canon* or the *Four Books of Confucianism* (四書):
  - *The Great Learning* (大學)
  - *The Doctrine of the Mean* (中庸)
  - *Analects* (論語)
  - *Mencius* (孟子)
- *Mohist Doctrines* (墨學)
- *Nei Jing* or *Yellow Emperor's Canon of Internal Medicine* (內經/黃帝內經)
- *Sheung Shu* (尚書)
- *Shijing* or *Book of Odes* (詩經)
- *Book of Rites* or *Li Ki* (禮記)
- *Zuo Zhuan* (左傳)
- *Historical Record* (史記)

References are also drawn from texts by modern Chinese scholars, and from English translations with commentary. These texts are replete with humanistic teachings, philosophical teachings, deep human passion and action.

Chinese culture and humans

Culture is a unique human phenomenon, constituted by the accumulated efforts and activities of human progress. The word 'culture' (in Chinese writing 文化, pronounced as wenhua), first appeared in *I Ching*, one of the oldest surviving Chinese classics, around 3000–4000 BCE. Here the word 'human' becomes part of a critical element in culture. In the *Bi* hexagram ☰☰ (chapter 22 of *I Ching*) is the following reflection on culture (my translation):

By observing the ceremonies/ornaments and regulations of people, we know human progress in this world 觀乎人文，以化成天下.

(Tang 2005:70)

Ceremonies and ornaments are signs of human prosperity and group activities. Regulations are essential for guiding human conduct toward formulating a peaceful society. However, while ceremonies and ornaments should be used appropriately, the inner qualities are more important than external appearances (Chow 2005). A more modern interpretation of culture embraces diverse knowledge and a holistic approach (Chan 1994:6, my translation):

> Culture is the results of human efforts, expressed materially or spiritually in religion, philosophy, law, politics, economics, tradition, ceremonies, science and arts. All these disciplines help to improve the qualities of individual life and societies as a whole.

The power of culture resides in the unifying force that binds an individual or a nation within the same culture. At the same time, we should be aware of the many different cultures in this world, and none is more significant than another.

Indeed, cultures can be communicated. How? We can learn from universal truths. For example, when writing about a subject an author applies his or her particular feelings and knowledge to express a particular truth. If the readers find the author's expression true in similar contexts, the author's truth may become universal truth and thus an objective phenomenon (Mau 2005).

The universal truths of a culture may derive from its core values, the foundation stones that provide the directions for people to follow. Core values can be timeless. Sun (2004) points out that in Chinese culture, the longest continuous culture in the world, the core values have endured unchanged. Some of these core values which inextricably link humans with Chinese culture will now be identified. Note that the word 'human' has a specific meaning in this book, which will continue to be explored throughout.

Development of humanistic philosophy

Before we consider the great tradition of humanism in Confucianism, Taoism and Mohism, it is essential to reflect on the historical context in which humanism emerged.

In ancient China, it was the Zhou dynasty (1122–221 BCE) that paved the way for the humanistic spirit. Prior to that, in the Shang dynasty (1700–1122 BCE) a widely held belief was that people and God were not separate; people prayed to various gods in nature. However, during the Zhou dynasty, the book *Li Ki* (*Book of Rites*) recorded the importance of people rather than God in the new dynasty: 'Shang people worshipped and served God, so God took priority before ceremonial etiquette. Zhou dynasty, instead, observed ceremonial etiquette and was generous in giving and far away from believing in spirits and God' (Lau 1978:18).

Humanism was reflected in *Shijing* (the *Book of Odes*), especially in the 40 hymns and eulogies. The first 305 poems were complied around the time when Zhou Kung (a great leader) assisted the government. *Shijing* states that it was during this period that the Zhou rulers were called the 'son of heaven' under the doctrine of the 'mandate of heaven', which means the rulers were given divine rights as long as they considered the welfare of the people. This increased emphasis on people was reinforced by the Zhou leaders, namely Zhou Kung, who advocated morality and humanism. Based on a concern for people and a spirit of humanism, he established ceremonies to be observed and songs for sacrifices to ancestors that contributed to a peaceful society for several hundred years.

The humanistic spirit had far-reaching consequences during the following Spring and Autumn Period (770–470 BCE) and the Warring States Period (475–221 BCE), the time of the birth of Confucianism, Taoism and Mohism. The Spring and Autumn Period and the Warring States Period were marked by an unprecedented liberation in intellectual thinking and changes in society as the feudal system declined. On the positive side, knowledge was no longer confined to the nobles, and ordinary people had greater opportunities to be exposed to learning. This exposure stimulated considerable progress in ideas and writing, notably in philosophy, history and literature (Fu 1975).

However, the other side of the picture was marked by devastation and deprivation, punctuated by battles, widespread social upheaval, political unrest, and uncertain existence. Territories were invaded and seized. Change was dramatic; during the Spring and Autumn Period there were more than 100 countries, but in the Warring States Period only seven remained (Fu 1975). At the same time, morality was disregarded as followers killed rulers and sons killed fathers. Mencius, a great ancient Chinese philosopher, lamented: 'there are no righteous wars in Spring and Autumn dynasty' (*Tsin Sin*, part 2, chapter 2).

In spite of the uncertainty and turmoil of these periods, Confucianism,

Taoism, and Mohism flourished, and people felt the need for a peaceful society governed by humanism. Confucius admired Zhou Kung and the Zhou period (1027–221 BCE) when it was at the height of its glory. He often dreamt of Zhou Kung, even noting in the *Analects* (chapter 7, verse 5) 'for a long time I have not dreamt of the Duke of Zhou'.

In Confucianism, humanism is glorified and practised as *yen* or 'benevolence'. As for Taoism, the whole book of the *Tao Te Ching* is replete with human equality, nature, and moral teaching. Humanism is reflected in the Mohists' ethics on political ideals, human relations, and education, in particular in Mozi's *Doctrine of Universal Love*.

The development of humanism was influenced by China's agricultural environment. China is predominately an agricultural country, with its earliest agricultural activities originating along the Yellow River. Agriculture started before the Shang dynasty, yet developed and became the main means of production during the Zhou dynasty. Early in the Zhou dynasty, the people's agricultural knowledge came from experience handed down from ancestors, personal experience with the geographical environment, and tribes whom they had conquered or with whom they interacted. At that time, agriculture was intrinsic in the lives of the people and their worshipping activities (Lau 1978).

This agricultural experience contributed significantly to the development of the humanistic spirit in Chinese culture. Humans and nature are closer in agricultural societies (Hui 1994), which are generally characterised by being more peaceful and stable because of the need to look after the land, to work together for production, and to take a practical worldview. In agricultural societies, life is largely directed by nature and the seasons. The people tend to be more inwardly directed, hard-working and respecting toward nature; to treasure long-term human relationships; and to have acquired an artistic view (Wai 1994; Tang 2005).

The agricultural environment also helps to develop a harmonious worldview and to refine one's character. Many enduring poems have been produced in tranquil agricultural environments. The metaphors of 'water' and 'hill' are used to symbolise wise and virtuous people in the *Analects* (Book 6, chapter 21). Note that the quiet environment of the hills helps to shape one's character as well as promote longevity:

The wise find pleasure in water; the virtuous find pleasure in hills. The wise are active, the virtuous are tranquil. The wise are joyful, the virtuous are long-lived.

Humanism in Confucianism

Humanistic spirit is realised in *yen*, 'benevolence', the highest virtue in Confucian teachings as exemplified in the *Analects* (attributed to Confucius). The concept of benevolence is all embracing and has diverse meanings in various contexts. The roots of benevolence are filial piety towards parents (chapter 1, verse 2). Filial piety is extended to include all elders, the living and the dead. Outside the family, benevolence includes the love of all mankind (chapter 12, verse 21) as all people are considered brothers in the world (chapter 12, verse 5). The power of benevolence helps to maintain an emotional balance which frees people from anxiety (chapter 9, verse 28). It is also believed that those who have benevolence can equally endure adversity and enjoy life; as such they can distinguish love and hate (chapter 4, verses 2 and 3).

The understanding of benevolence is gained through practice and is channelled through self and through relations with others. For the former, benevolence is initiated through conquering self (chapter 12, verse 1), by being cautious and slow in speech (chapter 11, verse 3), by living gracefully (chapter 13, verse 1), by being firm, enduring, simple, and modest (chapter 13, verse 27). For the latter, consideration for others becomes the basis of humanism (chapter 12, verse 2). Other qualities include loyalty and trustfulness (chapter 7, verse 24; chapter 13, verse 1) and the five practices of courtesy, tolerance, trustworthiness, quickness and generosity (chapter 17, verse 6). Moreover, for the sake of benevolence one can even sacrifice self (chapter 15, verse 8) as expressed in the following passage, which has become the hallmark of humanistic action:

> Men with aspiration and men with benevolence do not sacrifice benevolence to remain alive, but would sacrifice themselves for benevolence.

The Confucian scholar Mencius contributed to humanism with his recommendations for benevolent government and kind concern for others. Mencius said 'everyone can be the kings Yeos and Shuns' (*Kao Tsze*, part 2, chapter 2). Mencius is implying, firstly, that the success these two kings experienced in their personal lives as well as in political government was due to their moral integrity; and secondly, that people can learn from their examples and can similarly succeed if they try their best. Mencius famously declared that 'benevolence' means 'human heart' (*Kao Tsze*, part 1, chapter 11) and the 'love of mankind' (*Li Lau*, part 2, chapter 18) because good people have benevolence in their hearts, together with 'righteousness, propriety, and knowledge':

Benevolence, righteousness, propriety, and knowledge are not infused into us from without. We are certainly furnished with them...

(*Kao Tsze*, part 1, chapter 6, trans. Legge 1998:402)

Benevolence, in Mencius, was also realised through respect for the elderly and care for the young. Believing that people are inherently good, Mencius said that people have compassion and cannot tolerate the suffering of others (*Kung-sun Chau*, part 1, chapter 6, verse 2). Compassion was demonstrated by the example of a child about to fall into a well, a sight which would cause distress to all humans:

It is a feeling common to all mankind that they cannot bear to see others suffer... I say all men have such feelings because, on seeing a child about to fall into a well, everyone has a feeling of horror and distress... Not to feel distress would be contrary to all human feeling.

(*Kao Tsze,* part 1, chapter 7)

Humanism in Mohism

Humanism in Mohism was represented by its founder, Mozi (墨子), in his care and kind concern for people. He was dissatisfied with the unfair phenomena prevalent at that time (Warring States Period 475–221 BCE 戰國時代): all those who killed would be put to death, yet war was gloried; stealing domestic items was condemned, yet attacking others was rewarded. In addition, there was great disparity between the rich and the poor, and employment opportunities were based on family lines (Fu 1975). Moreover, he strongly opposed the human-imposed calamities that hindered humanity, including the strong oppressing the weak, the majority attacking the minority, the powerful manipulating the disadvantaged, the violence of men in using weapons to injure others. Mozi maintained that the roots of human conflicts sprang from human selfishness and the inability to love.

He proposed to satisfy three basic needs of people: to feed the hungry, to clothe the cold, to rest the tired. Moreover, Mozi summarised humanism in the chapter 'universal love' (兼愛) in which he explicitly described his care for the lives of people. The Chinese writing 兼 represents a person holding two grains, which implies caring for others on the basis of equal love (Sun 1999). Mozi expressed the belief that:

The major calamities in the world come from the failure of men to love one another, and hence can only be solved through the doctrine of universal love. The practice of universal love not only benefits the one who is loved, but also the one who loves, on the principle of reciprocity.

(Fung 1983:94)

There are two noteworthy messages here: 'benefit' and 'reciprocity'. A distinguishing feature of Mozi's doctrine was the principle of benefit (利), as in doing something that is good for the country and the people, which set the general standard in humanism. For example, Mozi opposed activities that wasted resources and thus limited benefit, such as military aggression (which was very expensive to maintain, destroying productivity), extravagant burial and music ceremonies (which took time away from productive work), and belief in fatalism (which promoted laziness and took away the drive to work hard). The task of humanity is to benefit the world and maximise utility. Humanity is further defined (*Mozi*, Book 25, 'Thrift in Funerals') as the positive outcomes of practising moral standards that 'can enrich the poor, multiply the few, secure those in danger, and set to order what is in disorder' (quoted from the Stanford Encyclopedia of Philosophy 2002).

Mozi also spoke of the principle of reciprocity, proposing that relationships based on consideration for others would benefit both sides, and could be applied at all levels: 'the kindness on the part of the ruler, the loyalty on the part of the ruled, of affection on the part of the father, and of filial piety on the part of the son' (Fung 1983:91).

Another area in which to realise humanity, according to Mozi, was education. Mozi believed that the goodness or badness of human nature was not determined by one's birth, but rather by one's environment. No doubt, Mozi's own actions as a teacher would have reflected humanism. He encouraged students to participate in persuasion and discussion, and to involve themselves in productive and educational activities. Logical thinking, scientific reasoning, and exploration using practical skills were characteristically emphasised in Mozi's humanism (Sun 1999). Mozi's thinking embraced moral integrity and scientific spirit, which was indeed advanced for his time.

Mohism is considered to be more thorough than Confucianism in its approach to humanism. Confucius emphasised 'benevolence' within a framework of hierarchy and aristocratic order (such as in family relationships and teaching), which Mozi called 'preferential care' (Sun 1999). Mozi taught the principle of 'universal love' that is all embracing and encourages equality in all human relationships, providing a rational foundation that unified the philosophy of humanism (Fung 1983:84).

Humanism in Taoism

Humanism in Taoism is reflected in its commitment to the preservation of life. The love of life as shown in the saying: 'Our life is our own possession, and its benefit to us is very great' (Fung 1948: 63). One's life is in one's hands and there is always something one can do about it. This positive attitude translates into the valuing of self and the need to continue to practise and make progress in order to attain self-excellence. Tao advocates the unity of humans and nature; underlying this principle is the ideal of harmonious relationships on earth – not going to extremes, taking the 'middle way' as the way to preserve life. Anything in this world that is too good or too bad may affect one's social relationships and health. A chapter in *Chuang Tzu* (399–295 BCE) provides evidence of this doctrine of the 'middle way' (Fung 1948:64):

> When you do something good, beware of reputation;
> When you do something evil, beware of punishment;
> Follow the middle way and take this to be your constant principle.
> Then you can guard your person, nourish your parents, and complete your
> natural term of years.

Moreover, in the process of practising Taoism, we learn to open up our minds and ourselves regarding the people around us. Taoist teaching encourages self-improvement and kind concern for other people as shown in *Tao Te Ching* (chapter 10, Chung 2004). The dedication of self in the Tao ennobles us so that out of love for humanity we can even dedicate our lives for the benefit of the world (chapter 13). Note Mencius held a similar view about self-sacrifice for benevolence. The practice of morality, as advocated in Taoism, is enduring and equally applicable for the self, for the family, for the state, for the country, and for the world (chapter 54). Non-action is a form of self-discipline expressed as a moral action. Freedom and equality are two of the main themes underpinning the concept of non-action, and hence the Tao is strongly against violence and war. The violent imposition of rules destroys the trust of the people (*Tao Te Ching*, chapter 31, trans. Lau 1963):

Sharp weapons are inauspicious instruments, everyone hates them. Therefore the man of the Way is not comfortable with them.

Those for whom victory is sweet are those who enjoy killing. If you enjoy killing, you cannot gain the trust of the people.

Instead of force, Taoist teaching (*Tao Te Ching*, chapter 46, trans. Lau 1963) suggests self-contentedness as a guard against human conflict, because many conflicts stem from greed:

Natural disasters are not as bad as not knowing what enough is.
Loss is not as bad as wanting more.
Therefore the sufficiency that comes from knowing what is enough is an eternal sufficiency.

The Taoist principles of mutual respect and of accepting difference whilst maintaining one's own identity are suggested (*Tao Te Ching*, chapter 61) for dealing with relationships between countries. In short, humanism of Taoism is manifested in the love of life, consideration for others, mutual respect, justice, equality, self-improvement, the preservation of life, and the rejection of war and violence. These are the ways of Tao.

The Chinese philosophical root of humanism – co-existence in harmony and balance – is inseparable from the concept of *yin* and *yang*, the basic principle informing Traditional Chinese Medicine. *Yin* and *yang* was described and explored in three of the greatest of the Chinese classics: *I Ching*, *Nei Jing* and *Tao Te Ching*, as follows.

Harmony and balance in humanism

The concept of *yin* and *yang* is a fundamental tenet of traditional Chinese philosophy, underlying how the phenomenon of life is thought to function in relation to the environment. This inseparability of microcosm and macrocosm is based on the traditional Chinese belief in the harmony of nature between heaven, earth and humankind, as expounded in Taoism and Confucianism. The *yin/yang* concept was formulated in *I Ching* (*The Book of Changes*) and further developed in the first Chinese medical classic, *Nei Jing* (*Yellow Emperor's Canon of Internal Medicine*), and in Taoist philosophy. An understanding of how the concepts of *yin* and *yang* are discussed in these texts is indispensable for understanding the concepts of balance and harmony in traditional Chinese culture and, through this, in Traditional Chinese Medicine.

I Ching (The Book of Changes)

I Ching provides the basic treatise on *yin* and *yang*. Around 700 BCE, *yin* and *yang* were referred to as 'the yielding', and 'the firm':

> Movement and rest have their definite laws; according to these *firm* and *yielding* lines are differentiated.

> (Baynes 1965:280)

The richly endowed meanings of *I Ching* are portrayed in the subtlety of natural order, social ideals, and human philosophy (Tang 2005). *I Ching* is characterised by the investigation of ideas and meanings through argument and debate, and the approach using graphic images or signs to explain the change phenomenon and relationships with other signs. In *I Ching*, heaven and earth are the source of all complicated natural and social phenomena, and they are based on *yin* and *yang*. As the *I Ching* says, 'one *yin* and one *yang* means Tao (the way)' (Tang 2005:13).

Yin and *yang* are described by symbolic lines in the sixty-four six-line diagrams called 'hexagrams'. The solid line (—) represents *yang*, heaven; and the broken line (– –) represents *yin*, the earth. *Yang*, heaven, refers to strength, movement and the positive and bright side of all things; *yin*, earth, represents receptiveness, quietness, darkness, and gentleness. All changes in natural phenomena operate in the ceaseless motion and complementarity of *yin* and *yang*, like heaven and earth, sun and moon.

I Ching was written three thousand years ago, and is one of the oldest surviving Chinese classics. The Emperor of the Qin Dynasty (221–207 BCE) ordered the burning of all ancient Chinese literature except books on 'medicine, divination, and husbandry'. *I Ching* survived because it included material on divination (Muller 1966). Apart from being the book of an oracle, it was regarded as a 'Book of Wisdom' (Baynes 1965). The two great Chinese philosophers, Confucius (551–479 BCE) and Lao Tzu (600–400 BCE), held the *I Ching* in high esteem. The *Analects* (Book 7, chapter 16) describes Confucius's regret about not devoting enough time to the study of *I Ching*. Regarding the perfection of himself, he said, 'If some years were added to my life, I would give fifty to the study of the *Yi* [*I Ching*], then I might come to be without great faults'. For Lao Tzu, the book inspired many of his maxims and teachings as reflected in the way of the Tao and the universal laws governing one's life.

A physician in the Ming Dynasty (1368–1644 CE), Cheung Gaai Bun (張介賓), stated his view of the importance of *I Ching* and of *yin* and *yang* to Traditional Chinese Medicine (my translation): 'If you do not know *I Ching*, you cannot be a great doctor', and again, 'the way of heaven and earth is based on *yin* and *yang*; the way of humans is made of *yin* and *yang*. Traditional Chinese Medicine and *I Ching* come from the same source, and articulate a philosophy of change' (Yiu 1984:38).

Nei Jing

Many chapters in *Nei Jing* (Tang Dynasty, 618–907 CE), the first Chinese medical classic, are explicitly devoted to the *yin* and *yang* correspondences between man and the environment, and provide information on the function of *yin* and *yang* and guidelines for prosperous and declining energies. Divided into two parts (*Plain Questions* and *Spiritual Pivot*), *Nei Jing* was written in the form of a dialogue between the Yellow Emperor and Qibo, a Taoist master. The Yellow Emperor raised a series of questions on matters of health and illness, and asked about ways to preserve health and prevent illness.

Yin and yang were perceived to be the originators and principles of all things, as noted in the texts: '*yin* and *yang* are the ways of heaven and earth', '*yin* and *yang* are the guiding principles of all things', '*yin* and *yang* are the parents of variations' (*Plain Questions*, chapter 5:31). Throughout the book we glimpse the duality of *yin* and *yang*: *yin* is earth, water, motionless, calm, turbid, cold, visible substance; *yang* is heaven, fire, movement, lucid, hot, and invisible refined energy. *Yin* and *yang* are dynamic and inter-related; however when *yin* and *yang* are given gendered qualities, this can imply that *yin* and *yang* perform fixed, specific roles. This binary perspective contrasts with the key original aspects of *yin* and *yang* – infinite change, and co-existence and complementarities in spite of differences.

The concept of the co-existence of *yin* and *yang*, discussed in *Nei Jing* (*Plain Questions*, chapter 66) is the crucial element of *yin* and *yang*. The creation of energy requires the constant interplay of *yin* and *yang*; without *yin*, the heavenly energy, *yang*, will not be able to descend; while without *yang*, the earthly energy, *yin*, will not be able to ascend.

Tao Te Ching

Tao contributes to the *yin* and *yang* balance, and thus preventive medicine, based on the principle of unity of body and spirit. Two holistic principles underlie this relationship. Firstly, the cultivation of self is governed by the unity of body and spirit, as reflected in the opening question in chapter 10 of *Tao Te Ching*: 'the spirit and the body are one, can you keep them from parting?' (trans. Cleary 1998). Secondly, underlying the self practice in body and spirit is the principle of the unity of humans and nature, the way of Tao (chapter 25). When one embraces nature and attains a purity of spirit, together with a body of vital energy, a healthy balance is achieved. This vital energy incorporates the *yin* and *yang*, as expressed in *Tao Te Ching* (chapter 42, trans. Lau 1963):

> The myriad creatures carry on their backs the *yin* and embrace in their arms the *yang* and are the blending of the generative forces of the two.

According to the philosophy, all things are comprised of *yin* and *yang*, and *qi*, the vital energy, is produced when the two forces combine. The traditional Chinese position of adherence to the natural order, of maintaining harmony in accord with nature but not to control it, is said to be one of the key differences from Western attitudes (Yu 1994). The naturalism of Tao and of *yin* and *yang* and the social harmony that arises from these principles contributed to early Traditional Chinese Medicine thinking and practice. Tao provides a code of conduct. Taoists believe that people's behaviours are ultimately responsible for their health and longevity (Jewell 1982).

Dynamic and ever-changing

The concept of change is a significant feature in the three above classics, in traditional Chinese culture, and in Traditional Chinese Medicine. Change is one of the main characteristics of *I Ching*, and is described as (my translation) 'up and down without constancy, the interchange of firm and yielding, and being adaptive to change' (Yiu 1984:42). This refers to constant change in the movements of heaven and earth, as with the interaction of *yin* and *yang*. Confucius reflected on this ceaseless phenomenon of change. Standing by a river and watching the constant flow of water (a metaphor for change on earth, and the transience of human life), Confucius exclaimed: 'It passes on just like this, not ceasing day or night' *(Analects*, Book 9, chapter 16). Change is constant, natural, and cyclical. As the *I Ching* says: 'Because of its changes and its continuity, it corresponds to the four seasons' (Baynes 1965:302). This change relationship between *yin* and *yang* is echoed in *Nei Jing* (*Plain Questions*, chapter 66:312): 'Under the interaction of heaven and earth, motion and motionless, up above and down below and the interlacing of *yin* and *yang*, changes will occur'. Tao also embraces the dynamic change of *yin* and *yang*. The understanding of the change relationship is critical to our thinking and provides us with new visions without cementing our ideas into impermeable binaries.

'The division of one into two' speaks of the continuous transformation of one force into others, as in the way of Tao described in *Tao Te Ching* (chapter 42): 'the way begets one, one begets two, two begets three; three begets the myriad of creatures'. The transformation of *yin* and *yang* corresponds to the processes of nature, which are manifested in the transformation of one force to the next.

The duality of *yin* and *yang* is dynamic. *Yin* and *yang* do not exist in a balanced state in the environment or in the body, but rather they oppose each other. As a result of this dynamism, *qi* (energy) is formed.

These overarching concepts of natural order and the need to keep in harmony with *yin* and *yang* reveal the Tao's influence in Traditional Chinese Medicine. Tao maintains the philosophy of harmony between this world and beyond. The call to return to nature in the Tao offers hope and a social solution, and acts as a 'soothing balm' to the human soul in times of distress (Lin 1977:111). According to *Nei Jing* (chapter 5:31), all things are generated by the harmonious relationship of *yin* and *yang*: '*Yin* and *yang* are the foundations of [life] and [death], when *yin* and *yang* are harmonised, the spirit will emerge, so *yin* and *yang* are the mansions of the spirit.'

Human centredness in traditional Chinese culture

The emphasis on human life as the centre of Chinese culture has been well documented by modern Chinese scholars (Lam 1995; Mau 2005; Pong 1992, Qian 1993; Tang 2000; and Yu 1994). The essence of this human focus is the effort of trying one's best and putting one's whole heart in doing things in life, and the harmonious relationships of nature, society and humans. Dr Sun Yat-sen (1963), widely revered as the 'father of modern China' in China and Taiwan, dedicated all his forty years of public life to people. Even in his Will, he expressed his kind concern for the people of this world. He emphasised the importance of freedom and equality, of being aware of the outside world, and of establishing good connections within and outside nations. His vision of ideal government was 'of the people, by the people, and for the people' (Sun 1963:183). Underlying these 'three people ideals', he believed that good government can be achieved only by prioritising and caring for people.

Similarly, Mencius's (c. 371–289 BCE) concept of ideal government also centred on people, in order to gain their support. He famously put people first by saying (*Tsin Sin*, part 2, trans. Legge 1998:483):

> The people are the most important element in a nation; the spirits of the land and grain are the next; the sovereign is the slightest.

Other notable examples include the ancient Chinese scholar Luk Cheung Shan (陸象山) who elegantly declared, 'even if I don't know a word, I have to be a proper person' (Yu 1994:18). A 'proper person' means trying one's best in this world. *Sheung Shu* (尚書), the oldest Chinese historical book (2300–1000 BCE, recording the dynasties of Yu, Hsia, Shang, and Zhou, proposes 'using moral disciplines to improve human lives' (正德 利用 厚生) (Mu 1988:3; Pong 1992:59). The concept centres on the relations between self and self, and between self and others – to be strict and conquer self, and to be lenient toward others. It also implies that one has to refine self first in order to help others.

Humans are relational and have profound social significance in the Chinese sense. The word 'human' (in Chinese writing 人, and pronounced as ren) refers to three relationships: with self, with others, and with the universe. Underlying these relationships is harmonious co-existence.

With self

'Self' is the focal theme for attaining self-excellence in many Chinese classics. This is exemplified in *The Great Learning* (c. 400 BCE), which is generally attributed to Confucius:

> The principle of learning is to glorify and to develop our true moral nature, to effect good change, and to arrive at our very best conditions.
>
> (*The Great Learning*, chapter 1, Yeung 2004:166–167, my translation)

The two themes indicated in the message above are 'our true moral nature' and 'our very best conditions'. In Confucianism, human nature is considered to be good (essentially the basic view of Mencius, who earned the title of 'Second Sage' after Confucius). Our true moral self should be guided by 'benevolence, righteousness, filial piety, loyalty, and forgiveness' (Yeung 2004:166), attributes which come from our inner self. It is important, therefore, to uncover our moral self and to develop our best condition, unclouded by the complications of worldly affairs. In the *Analects*, 'our best condition' (止於至善) can be realised by practising 'benevolence by the leaders, respect by the juniors, filial piety by children, kindness by parents, and trust between countries' (*Analects*, chapter 4).

Significantly, *The Great Learning* (chapter 1) maintains that the basis for all these practices comes from refining one's character, and is equally applicable to all levels of people: 'from the Son of Heaven down to the mass of people, all must consider the cultivation of self the root of everything'. The expansion of self essentially embodies the social responsibility that contributes to world peace, as reflected in the saying 'self cultivation assists in regulating one's family, governing a state, and pacifying the world' (身修而後家齊，家齊而後國治，國治而後天下平).

In *The Book of Changes* or *I Ching*, self is positively associated with continuous striving for improvement (chapter 1, Ch'ien / *Creative* hexagram ䷀). In this image, the powerful heavenly body moves ceaselessly. The implication is that one should cultivate a strong spirit and a good character, through which one will be able to influence others. If one has secured a sound foundation, one can confront danger and act with courage and confidence, and this is viewed as a noble act (chapter 29, *K'an / Abysmal (Water)* hexagram ䷜). As Mencius says, in difficult times true human nature, wisdom and knowledge are often revealed (Chow 2005). In other situations, one tends to lose sight of balance when one has power (chapter 34, *Ta Chuang / Power of the Great* hexagram ䷡). The issue of control is elaborated on later (chapter 60, *Chieh / Limitation* hexagram ䷻), regarding the importance of adhering to nature by acting appropriately. Likewise, the ability to control self is considered 'real strength' which will produce positive outcomes such as justice and righteousness, whereas controlling others by using force will not produce these positive outcomes.

Behind this notion of self-discipline is the principle that we should be flexible and cautious and should act accordingly, that we should be guided by self-awareness. Moreover, appropriate actions are determined by time and space – 'when' one should stop and 'where' one should stop. All phenomena in nature are subjected to constant change, according to *The Book of Changes*. With self-awareness, we can exercise self-discipline, and act appropriately. As elaborated on in *I Ching*, (chapter 5, Tang 2005:84, my translation):

> Sometimes we take the top position, other times the lesser one. We change not because of wrong intentions in our hearts. Sometimes we advance,

other times we retreat, not because we are away from people. This is because we are trying to refine our self in order to grasp the right opportunity and act at the right time.

At the same time, self-discipline also means to prepare for a better future. Even in times of danger one should remain conscious of world affairs and help whenever possible.

Importantly, we should appreciate that *The Book of Changes* is not only about flexible change but also about what is unchanged. What really changes is the external phenomenon; the basic values deep inside do not change.

Zuo Zhuan (左傳), the earliest Chinese work of narrative history (covering the period 722–468 BCE), mentions three guiding principles for living life and leaving a meaningful legacy: 'to establish virtues, to establish contributions, and to establish knowledge' (立德, 立功, 立言). According to these principles, one should refine self, contribute to others and society, and give helpful advice and share knowledge (Mu 1988). Qian (2004) suggests that by means of practising these principles, people can 'live on' after their deaths because their contributions survive in people's hearts.

The teachings of Confucius highlight the importance of learning and self-discipline. Regarding learning, Confucius emphasised positive self-improvement in this present life by engaging self in whatever one does and in the best way one can. In the *Analects* (chapter 1), the pleasure of learning through regular practice is noted. Speech must be congruent with action, therefore practice is a critical part of the process, involving listening, speaking, observing, and acting (chapter 2, verse 18). In addition, it is important to learn extensively, to question enthusiastically, and to reflect upon self (chapter 19, verse 6). The devotion to learning is shown in remembering, self-awareness, and reflection (chapter 19, verse 5):

> Every day to acknowledge what is lacking, and every night not to forget what one has acquired. This can be called devotion to learning.

On the other hand, self-discipline is the prerequisite for attaining 'benevolence', which Confucius and Mencius strongly emphasised is to be practiced with the utmost strength. Moreover, the *Analects* (chapter 12, verse 1) points out that the fulfilment of benevolence depends on self and not on others:

> To discipline self to fulfil the rites is benevolence... the practice of benevolence originates from self and not from others.

Other guidelines include to conduct self-examination three times a day (chapter 1, verse 4), and to be strict on self and lenient towards others (chapter 15, verse 14). These self-disciplines take courage and confidence and imply conquering self to provide the basis of virtue and building blocks toward self-excellence and self-expansion. In unfavourable conditions, however, one should display determination and perseverance (chapter 4, verse 5), and should be the first to face difficulties and the last to think of rewards (chapter 6, verse 20).

For Mencius, it is the heart that guides the self, as stated in the famous dictum (*Tsin Sin*, part 1), 'one who puts in one's whole heart (with utmost effort) knows human nature'. Working with correct morals that arise from the heart, Mencius states that people will have great strength to produce just deeds. However, any act without conscience will deplete energy:

> It [physical vigour] is nurtured by rectitude; it remains unharmed and permeates the entire universe. The physical vigour in this sense is the fit recipient for Justice and the Way. Without it, man is ill-nourished... If an act of ours does not meet with approval in the heart, then vigour [the life-force] is ill-nourished.

> (*Mencius*, trans. Dobson 1963:86)

This heart is not limited to directing self alone but extends outside, embracing family, country, and the world, touching on virtually all one's life. Once again, such a high ideal of openness and unselfishness provides a fine example of Confucian 'benevolence'.

The founder of Mohism, Mozi (around 468–376 BCE, coming after Confucius and before Mencius) tried to distinguish human nature from the nature of animals. Mozi perceived that human survival requires active self-involvement in production. He advocated a humble life, discouraged extravagance, and emphasised education.

The *Tao Te Ching* (chapter 1) states self is the basis for achieving the Tao in accordance with nature, to achieve balance. Tao is described as an abstract concept that cannot be defined in words (道，可道，非常道，名，可名，非常名, 'The Tao that can be told is not the eternal Tao. The name that can be named is not the eternal Name.'). This quote provides the summary and the essence of the whole book about Tao. The explanation is that real Tao has no material form that we can grasp, but rather exists in a spiritual state, that is, in our hearts. Again, *Tao Te Ching* (chapter 21) describes the Tao in terms of various elements: 'as form, as thing, as essence, and as belief' (trans. Lau 1963). In spite of the vagueness and obscurity of the Tao, its elements can be understood through immersing oneself in the Tao. In other words, it is through individual experience and practice of Tao that one finds the true self, and thus the Tao (Masami 2005).

The water symbol is used repeatedly in *Tao Te Ching* (chapters 8, 43, and 78) to glorify the soft and gentle qualities which overcome the strong and the hard; the Tao benefits all things yet takes a humble position. For example (chapter 78) water, though soft and yielding, can win over adversity:

> Nothing in the world is as soft and yielding as water,
> Yet nothing can better overcome the hard and strong,
> For nothing can replace water.
> The soft overcomes the hard,
> The yielding overcomes the strong.

In the world we may tend to consider the strong as powerful and regard the other side as weak. However, the virtues of non-action (providing more autonomy and freedom for others), the natural order, equality, quietness, gentleness, and simplicity are highly preferred in Tao. For example, the way of Tao was demonstrated through preserving the vital force in a simple and quiet manner, as reflected in the texts of *Tao Te Ching* (trans. Lau 1963:298):

> You must be still; you must be pure; not subjecting your body to toil, not agitating your vital force... Watch over and keep your body, and all things will of themselves give it strength.

Other moral characters that one should adhere to include humbleness and unselfishness (chapter 7). Using the universe as an example, Taoism shows that heaven and earth are lasting (天長地久) because of their unselfishness and humbleness. In view of Tao, those who lower themselves will eventually get support from people and can be free from danger:

> Heaven and earth are enduring. They are enduring because they do not live for themselves.
>
> ... The sage places oneself behind people... and outside without selfishness and will obtain support and security.

In addition, understanding self is praised more highly than understanding others. Such a belief helps to elevate the spiritual self to be free from prejudice and greed and, importantly, to not go to extremes. Chapter 33 says 'to understand self is wise, to conquer self is mighty, and to be contented is rich'. In this chapter was emphasised the need to be self-aware, to overcome self-imposed limitations, and to be content with what one has.

The importance for self to maintain a sound mind that is quiet and stable, free from 'wishes', 'ambitions', 'fame' and 'gain,' is emphasised in *Nei Jing*. Turmoil in life, as suggested by the *Nei Jing* (*Plain Questions*, chapter1:8) undermines a sound mind:

> As [people]are having a quiet and stable state of mind, no desire can seduce their eyes, and no obscenity can entice their heart. Although the intelligence and moral character between different people are not the same, yet they can all attain the stage of giving no personal gain or loss.

With others

The human relationship with others is seen as the continuum of self. In Chinese culture the concept of 'Equilibrium and Harmony' (中和) is an indispensable and significant feature of this human relationship between self and others. This concept is constituted by two elements, one internal and one external. The internal element relates to an individual's subjective state; the external element is manifested in one's social relations and behaviour. According to *The Doctrine of the Mean* (chapter 2, notes by Yeung 2004), various human emotions such as 'pleasure, anger, sorrow, or joy', if not expressed, are viewed as the state of 'Equilibrium'; if expressed in the proper manner without extremes; they are called 'Harmony'. In Confucianism, harmony and equilibrium are the roots of refining conduct and morality; when actions are properly carried out, harmony prevails.

This harmonious relationship underlines each person's relations with others; the individual is considered as a role or a set of relations with others, never in isolation (Pong 1993). For instance, *I Ching* (chapter 38, *Khwei* hexagram ☲☱) denotes the principles of separation and union, differences and commonalities. These phenomena are seen to operate in a circle; after a long separation, there will be union. Therefore one should seek similarities among differences. It is important to accept differences while seeking commonalities based on mutual respect and trustfulness (Chow 2005). The attributes of trust and sincerity are also implied in other situations (chapter 45, *Zhui* hexagram ☱☷; chapter 46, *Shang* hexagram ☷☴) as the basic principles for group gatherings and work situations, such as promotion. In group interactions, one should be humble and direct one's energy for the group. For work purposes, one may need to seek help and advice from experienced and successful people. However, one should continue to work hard and not just depend on others, and one should maintain a harmonious relationship with the people from whom one seeks help (Chow 2005).

In Confucius's teaching, harmonious relationships in the family situation were translated into various roles exemplified by filial piety, which was defined in the *Analects* (Book 1, chapter 7) as the utmost strength to treat parents with reverence, and through which each member in the family dutifully carried out his or her role 'when the father is father, when the son is son' (chapter 11). Confucian teaching in filial piety also suggested it includes taking care of those who are in need of help, such as to look after children and parents. This obligation was reflected in the Confucian canon *Li Ki* or the *Book of Rites* (Dawson 1995:159):

> To exhaust his strength in discharging his service as a tribute of gratitude to his parents, he dares not but do his utmost.
>
> (*Li Ki,* Book 21, section I:4)

The encouragement to exert one's utmost strength in filial piety and learning was endorsed by Confucius's distinguished disciple, Tsze-hea. (On the death of his son, Tsze-hea wept himself blind, but survived to a good old age). Tsze-hea's view was that one demonstrated learning by serving one's parents as well as one could (together with two other virtues: serving seniors with devotion and friends with sincerity):

> In serving his parents, he can exert his utmost strength… although men say that he has not learned, I will certainly say that he has.

In the view of Mencius, trying one's best is filial piety. Mencius (*Tang Wan Kung,* part 1:252) suggests that the relation of filial piety is governed by a set of defining rules between seniors and juniors (*Mencius* section 252, trans. Legge 1998):

> Between father and son, there should be affection… between husband and wife, attention to their separate functions.

Moreover, the defining relationships between seniors and juniors are based on benevolence and righteousness (*Kao Tsze,* part 2, chapter 4). The harmonious family relationship is also echoed in *The Great Learning* (chapter 4 in Yeung's notes 2004). It is stated that when one can carry out one's duty according to Confucianism (namely, a son should exhibit filial piety, a father should show kindness) and glorify the traditions handed down, one is said to be living in harmony and to have realised one's potential. The binding relationship of father and son also serves to continue the family line.

As suggested earlier, filial piety is not confined to family relationships. Relations with others are extensions of filial piety, the one–big–family ideal of Confucianism. The relationship resembles a vertical line extending upwards with respect to seniors and parents and further, to ancestors and to the universe, and in the other direction with love toward those who are junior and below. Confucius advises us to be lenient and considerate toward others: 'don't do to others what you don't want others to do to you' (*Analects,* chapter 12). In practice, such ideals are shown in various situations: courtesy at home, respect at work and loyalty to other people (chapter 13), faithfulness at work and sincerity with friends (chapter 4), and trustfulness in speech (chapter 7).

Another aspect of the harmonious relationship is represented by concern for the body of others (Leung 2004; Sun 2004). In Sun's view, the emphasis on the body starts in the family where one learns caring for others, for example by inviting friends for dinner, offering gifts and money, helping friends to relax. In my findings on the meanings of Traditional Chinese Medicine (Leung 2004), Chinese people often use food to express care for the bodies of their family members and friends.

We glimpse Mozi's views on the relations of humans with others in his famous doctrine of 'universal love', a 'love' that permits no unfair treatment of others, as everyone should 'enjoy equally and suffer equally' (Fung 1948: 53). Moreover, the standard of universal love includes benefit to others as well as reciprocity, that is, consideration for others. He promoted social behaviour that was caring, considerate, and equal.

In Tao, equality prevails between self and others. Co-existence requires a positive attitude, openness, initiative and trustfulness, which all enhance relationships. In the non-dualistic position of Tao, commonalities and differences are part of the natural phenomenon and should be treated equally, such that co-existence is achievable. *Tao Te Ching* (chapter 2, trans. Lau 1963:6) states:

> The whole world recognises the beautiful as the beautiful, yet this is only the ugly;
>
> The whole world recognises the good as good, yet this is only the bad;

Thus something and nothing produces each other;
The difficult and the easy complement each other;
The long and the short offset each other;
The high and the low incline towards each other;
Note and sound harmonise each other;
Before and after follow each other.

The first two sentences state the opposing nature of things in binary terms, such as 'beautiful and ugly', 'good and bad', yet they are dependant on each other. In the following lines, examples are drawn from natural and social phenomena to explain their interrelationships and co-existence.

With the universe

There are two themes regarding the relationships of humans and the universe: the unity of humans and the universe, and the historical, social and cultural context of life and death. In the first place, humans and the universe are on friendly terms in traditional Chinese culture. The universe (or heaven) is not seen as having been created by God, nor are humans and the universe seen as separate in a way that humans cannot reach the position of God (Sun 2004). On the contrary, in Chinese culture the universe and humans are seen as one, operating in a harmonious relationship. The fusion of human and the universe is stated in *I Ching* (hexagram 22 ䷕), in that the objective universe and the subjective character of humans are linked (Tang 2005:69). *I Ching* describes the change between phenomena; for example, after the sunset will come the moonlight. The same occurs with the seasons – winter disappears and summer will return and so the seasons cycle continuously. If something has gone, it does not mean it will be gone forever, but simply that it is gone for now. Similarly, if something exists now, this does not imply it will exist permanently, but only that it exists at this time (Chow 2005).

The close relationship between humans and the universe is expressed in the following passage from *I Ching* (Tang 2005:57, 58, my translation). Note the parallel drawn between good people and the universe:

Heaven and earth have no hearts; therefore their greatest virtues are to nurture all things on earth. Good people have hearts; therefore their greatest virtues are benevolence and love; they can be aligned with the universe, and their brightness is equal to the heavenly stars.

In Taoism, all phenomena co-exist in the universe, including heaven, earth and people. Lao Tzu (600–400 BCE), advanced the idea that all phenomena on earth come from nature (chapter 25 of *Tao Te Ching,* 有物混成，先天地生，可以為天地母, trans. Legge 1998):

> There was something undefined and complete,
> coming into existence before Heaven and Earth.
> … It may be regarded as the Mother of all things.

This concept of 'enduring Heaven and Earth' as expressed earlier (*Analects,* chapter 7) also implies the oneness of the human and the universe. The non-dualistic relationships of naturalness, equal standing, and balance in the life-world permeate the text of *Tao Te Ching.* The Tao's cosmological vision of nature operates in an spontaneous, endless, circular manner, and phenomena are relative and relational. According to Chuang Tzu (399–295 BCE), a distinguished thinker regarding the Tao, the oneness of human with universe is illustrated by 'levelling all things' as 'heaven and earth are together with me, I and all things are One' (Chu and Wong 2003:37). In the same chapter, Chuang Tzu's dream of a butterfly provides another example. He could not distinguish a butterfly from himself, or which was real; 'Chuang the I' was the object and the butterfly was the subject. Yet in the non-dualistic world of Tao, object and subject are one, transcending the boundaries of space and time. That is the way of Tao.

In the Han Dynasty (206 BCE – 220 CE), a holistic view of the system of the universe was established. Humans were perceived as part of the universe and not separate from it: 'If we move one hair we move the whole body' (Hui 1994:50). Humans were not perceived to transcend nature, but rather to co-exist with it, in unity, inseparable. Besides, nature had been imbued with deep human feelings; humans and the universe could communicate and were interchangeable. The ancient Chinese scholar, Luk Cheung Shan, expressed it this way: 'the universe is the same as my heart, and my heart is the same as the universe' (Wai 1972:128). Symbolic expressions of the connectedness of humans and the universe can be found in many poems about nature, such as the poems of Tao Yuan-ming (陶淵明, 365–427 BCE). His identity with nature is richly depicted in one of his popular poems (Hermitary 2002):

> I built my hut within where others live, but there is no noise of carriages
> and horses.

You ask how this is possible: when the heart is distant, solitude comes.
I pluck chrysanthemums by the eastern fence, and see the distant southern mountains.
The mountain air is fresh at dusk, flying birds return in flocks.
In these things there lies a great truth, but when I try to express it, I cannot find the words.

The poem highlights the unity of human and nature; transcending time, human and nature are merged into one. The poet was able to appreciate the beauty of nature because he could remain solitary and project his image into nature.

According to Wai (1972), this belief in the unity of humans with the universe contributes to the harmonious relationships and deep human feelings which inspired many poets and writers to produce some of the finest scholarship. At the same time, in ancient days it discouraged interest in scientific research.

On the other hand, the unity of humans and the universe is also influenced by the focus of life orientated to the present. This orientation has been influenced by ancient thinking about the matters of life and death, that we should direct our energy toward this present world.

According to Confucius, 'If you do not understand life, how can you understand death?' (*Analects*, chapter 11). Confucian thinking centres on the present world: to live is more important than to die. This attitude had great impact on later dynasties. For example, in the early Qin Dynasty (221–207 BCE), the meaning of death was conveyed by the metaphor of 'the light went out' (Lam & Wong 1995:62). The view of death held during the Song (960–1279) and Ming Dynasties (1368–1644 CE) emphasised the cultivation of ideal characters in this present world, but not pursuing longevity (Fung 1973).

In the view of Lao Tzu, as expressed in *Tao Te Ching*, death was as much a part of nature as life, as reflected in the opening sentence of chapter 50: 'Exiting life, we enter death'. Moreover, Lao Tzu pointed out that three out of ten people would live long, and three out of ten people would die early. These two types of people all die naturally without regret. Yet there is another type: three out of ten people are too worried about death and are restless. They die early because they are against nature. The explanation is that people who try to differentiate between life and death, not considering them as a whole, would come to fear death, lose their sense of calmness, and therefore die early.

Life and death, in the view of Chuang Tzu (399–295 BCE), is simply an existing state; moving from one state to the other is a natural change and a natural phenomenon in the universe. He distinguished people who adhere to nature as real people in his *Great Teacher of the Source* (*Inner Chapter* section). For them, life and death are part of nature, like night and day, therefore the beginning and the end of life are equally good. Unaffected by life and death, one shows detachment from life, and from this point one is able to open up and transcend time (Cleary 1993:108):

> Once he was detached from life, he was able to penetrate clearly… he was able to see the unique… he could transcend time… he was able to enter into the birthless and deathless.

Many of the poems of Tao Yuan-ming (365–427 BCE) embody his optimistic view of death and his adherence to nature. As he approached his own death, he wrote a touching poem to his son on the matter, saying 'life and death have their destiny, riches and prosperity are decided by Heaven' (Tao 2005:256, my translation). According to Tao Yuan-ming, when there is life, there is also death; therefore there is no need to fear death because it is part of nature, even 'to die young does not mean short life' (Tao 2005:220). His views on life and death were also reflected in three poems written as dialogue between the 'Body' and the 'Shadow', and the analytical 'Soul' which listened to their views on life and death. Body said that heaven and earth, mountain and river were everlasting, yet the human form must die and disappear, and suggested that humans should make use of the lifetime to drink more wine. Shadow held a different view, proposing that humans should do more charitable work instead of drinking wine for pleasure. Listening to the views of Body and Shadow, Soul analysed that drinking wine would shorten one's life and that doing charitable work might not be appreciated, that life and death were part of nature and so humans should take things easy. This poet was saying that fear of death stems from worrying too much about our body. If we consider body and soul as one, such that when the body ends so does the soul, we can be free from worry.

Value of Chinese cultural core values in the modern world

In current times we are seeing the disturbing phenomena of massive human conflicts and destruction among nations – racial discrimination, religious wars, testing of nuclear weapons, environmental pollution, unchecked use of chemicals, fake medicines, and much more.

We are not at peace on the individual level either. We are beset by alarming news of domestic violence, drug addiction, child abuse, stealing and manipulation. Apart from the outward displays of human misbehaviour, inwardly individuals are experiencing insecurity, loss of identity, emotional imbalance, lack of trust and respect, selfishness, greediness, and self-centredness. Driven by the pursuit of power and excessive materialism, people have left behind important human values that uphold the individual and cement human relationships.

What we need now is peace and harmony within us as individuals, in society and among nations. The core values embedded in Confucianism, Mohism and Taoism are practical and can be realised through action and practice. The advice for refining self includes the spiritual values of acting appropriately, trying one's best in the present world, developing self-reliance and self-understanding, continuously striving for improvement, being humble, being contented, and seeking simplicity. These values are not prevalent among people in the modern world, but they are values that help people to maintain inner balance and overcome self-imposed limitations.

By fully developing the self through the practice of benevolence, universal love, mutual respect, filial piety and trust, one is able to overcome human barriers and to establish a harmonious co-existence (seeking similarities while accepting differences) with others. Such an expansion of self, from within a family to the outside world, is truly humanistic. The practice of humanism embodies consideration for others, for one will tend to think less of oneself and will put other people first, and thus generate a sense of righteousness. Such unselfishness is essential for this modern world. Here I quote Mencius's precept on righteousness (*Mencius*, chapter 10): 'I like life, and I also like righteousness. If I cannot keep the two together, I will let life go, and choose righteousness'.

The Tao's non-dualistic view of freedom, receptiveness and equality, of avoiding war and violence through trust among nations, coupled with the Mohists' anti-war and anti-aggression ideals of equality and universal love, brought further together with the Confucian principle of benevolence as embodied by filial piety, compassion, trust and mutual respect, can contribute to world peace. I believe the spiritual and moral values of Chinese culture and its human centredness offer valuable insights and guiding principles in this unsettling modern world, and this offers us hope.

Reflections

Traditional Chinese culture has a long history of emphasising the importance of human lives; in particular the spiritual and moral dimensions mentioned in the Chinese classical studies. This understanding can be visualised as three interrelated layers.

At the centre of the surface layer are 'humans' guided by idealistic values, trying one's best in life, putting one's whole heart at work, and seeking harmonious co-existence with others.

The middle layer is composed of the three human relationships: with self, with others, and with the universe. These relationships reveal the core values of Chinese culture, as realised through practices and action. For self, good virtue can be fully developed by practising benevolence, righteousness, filial piety, appropriate action, self-discipline, self-reliance, humility, and continuous learning. The expansion of self embraces social responsibility in relationships with others, highlighting universal love, harmonious co-existence (seeking similarities and accepting differences) through mutual respect and trustfulness, equality, peace, and compassion. This non-dualistic relationship is defined by a belief in the oneness of humans and the universe, a belief that all phenomena are related and inter-related.

The influence of humanism is the layer that underlies the previous layers. Humanism is glorified and developed in the teachings of Confucius, Mozi and Tao. They share the same vision in the humanistic approach: self-improvement, respect, kind concern for others, harmonious co-existence, and the upholding of humanity even at the expense of self. Such unselfishness and consideration for others is truly humanistic.

In this chapter I have proposed applying the core values of traditional Chinese culture to the modern world, as a way of restoring individual inner balance and charting a way toward world peace. Leaving behind this study of traditional Chinese culture, we enter another phase in this book, the discussion of a study into the various meanings of Traditional Chinese Medicine held by Chinese people (and two Westerners) in Australia. I will present the concept of complementarity as illustrated in the next chapter, which is the first chapter presenting results. The positioning of Traditional Chinese Medicine in relation to Western medicine and concerns about the transmission of Traditional Chinese Medicine knowledge are raised.

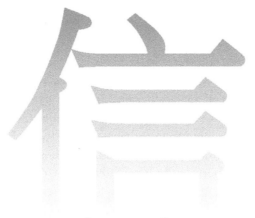

chapter three

Beliefs

(Pronounced as *xin*, which means 'beliefs' in health and human trust)

The best practice in health is Traditional Chinese Medicine and Western medicine complementing each other.

A 75-year-old man in Sydney,
originally from Mainland China

Introduction

Our understanding of disease and illness are socially and culturally constructed, and illness involves cultural practices and shared meanings arising from patients' lived experiences (Morris 1998). Research shows that much ill health never reaches medical attention, a phenomenon termed the 'illness iceberg' (Last 1963). Understanding lay beliefs and culture relating to health and illness is significant for health professionals delivering health care, particularly in preventive and early intervention services.

Kleinman and his colleagues (1978) proposed that lay knowledge was a valuable diagnostic tool in the understanding of personal illness (Kleinman & Seeman 2000). Other researchers into health and illness have recognised the importance of lay knowledge for understanding disease and illness (Prior, Pang & Huat 2000), lay beliefs in health care (Furnham 1988; Mechanic 1992; Furnham 1994; Nettleton 1995; Siahpush 1999), social determinants of health (Duhl 1981), social meanings of alternative medicine (Pawluch, Cain & Gillett 2000), and the relevance of people's cultural beliefs about the causes of illness to their health-seeking behaviour (Lupton 1994; Ell & Castaneda 1998).

This chapter discusses findings about people's beliefs of Traditional Chinese Medicine in the areas of the relationships between Traditional Chinese Medicine and Western medicine, and the transmission of Traditional Chinese Medicine knowledge.

The participants

Forty-eight participants were interviewed regarding their experiences and conceptions of Traditional Chinese Medicine. All participants were Chinese apart from two Westerners (in Brisbane) who were included because of their close association with Traditional Chinese Medicine (in one case, the wife of a Chinese participant, and in the other case, a Chinese martial arts teacher with considerable familiarity with Traditional Chinese Medicine). Hong Kong was the birthplace of the largest number of participants (nineteen), followed by Mainland China (Beijing, See Yup and Shanghai) with twelve and Taiwan with seven. Five had been born in Papua New Guinea and three in Australia. Singapore and Vietnam were the birthplaces of one participant each. I conducted all the interviews myself, in one of four languages. Cantonese was used by the greatest number of participants (fourteen), followed by English (nine), Mandarin (seven), and See Yup dialect (six).

Participants belonged to three main age groups: young (15–30 years, thirteen participants), middle-aged (35–65 years, twenty-one participants), and elderly (68–87, fourteen participants). Across all participants and within each age group, the participants were divided roughly evenly between males and females. Thirty-six people were interviewed individually in Armidale, Sydney and Brisbane. The remaining participants were interviewed in two groups in Brisbane; one group was young people originally from Hong Kong, and the other group was middle-aged people originally from Taiwan.

Traditional Chinese Medicine and Western medicine

Participants in the present study did not rely solely on Traditional Chinese Medicine, which was consistent with considerable research into the use by Chinese people of Traditional Chinese Medicine in conjunction with Western medicine in Australia (Hage, Tang, Li, Lin, Chow & Thien 2001; Tang & Easthope 2000), the United States (Pang, Jordan-March, Silverstein & Cody 2003; Guo 2000), China (Harmsworth & Lewith 2001; Khng 2003), and Hong Kong (Chan, Mok, Wong, Tong, Day, Tang & Wong 2003).

Rather, participants in this study used Traditional Chinese Medicine alongside Western medicine, actively seeking the best of both worlds in order to meet their health needs. They were aware of the fundamental differences and complementary nature of these two medical models, and actively sought benefit and better quality health care from each.

Complementary use

Participants generally believed that Traditional Chinese Medicine and Western medicine enrich each other and that each has its own role to play. Western medicine was generally seen to offer quick pain relief, lower temperatures rapidly, be better for surgery, and have preferable taste and colour (particularly according to the younger participants). On the other hand, Traditional Chinese Medicine was preferred for chronic illness, had a reputation for fewer side effects, and was popular for long-term preventive and therapeutic purposes. These attitudes are illustrated in the comments of this 76-year-old man in Sydney (originally from See Yup, Mainland China):

> Western medicine provides a quick relief of pain, for example, 'pain due to wind'. I think the best medicine for elderly people is the integration of Traditional Chinese Medicine and Western medicine (中西結合). I use Western medicine for 'pain due to wind'; I use Traditional Chinese Medicine for 'pain in bones' and rheumatism.

> The 'wind' he referred to here describes a causative factor of illness, common traditional construct (discussed later in this chapter). However, for a more enduring pain – such as rheumatism, which he referred to as 'pain in bones' – Traditional Chinese Medicine was preferred.

A 75-year-old man in Sydney (originally from Mainland China) thought Western medicine was better for lowering the temperature in acute situations, but for long-term therapeutic purposes he chose Traditional Chinese Medicine. Each was considered to have its own merit:

> Western medicine is effective in lowering the temperature immediately. But 'strengthening our body and nourishing our energy' is the job of

Traditional Chinese Medicine. The best practice in health is that Western medicine and Traditional Chinese Medicine can complement each other. We cannot say which side is not good. For clinical practice such as surgery, Western medicine is better. In terms of treating inflammation, for proper healing, Traditional Chinese Medicine is better.

The younger-aged focus group in Brisbane (originally from Hong Kong) suggested Western medicine had better taste and colour, which appealed to them more, and that Western medicine was quicker and more convenient. A preference for the taste and colour of Western medicine could be explained by their early experiences with paediatric medicines in Hong Kong, which were sweet and colourful. Also Traditional Chinese Medicine would have been more accessible in Hong Kong, often in the form of ready-made herbal tea drinks, than in Brisbane where they now lived and where only a very small number of shops dealt in Traditional Chinese Medicine.

However, this group reported that Western medicine seemed to contain too many chemicals; chemotherapy also concerned them, because of the side-effects that can result in the loss of physical attractiveness. As a result, 'you do not know whether you will eventually look like a ghost or a human being'. In their culture of origin (Hong Kong), body image is an important social consideration.

An interesting counterpoint to this perception was voiced by the other Brisbane group (originally from Taiwan), who mentioned that one of the main problems with Traditional Chinese Medicine was that too many chemicals now contaminate Traditional Chinese Medicine herbs.

Another point that emerged from the interviews was that Western medicine was considered scientific in approach, whereas Traditional Chinese Medicine was considered more intuitive. While Western medicine was considered to be very narrow in its focus and application, Traditional Chinese Medicine was viewed as reassuringly holistic by a 39-year-old man in Armidale (originally from Shanghai, Mainland China):

Western medicine is faster in healing. Yet it only looks after a small part. When you have headache, Western medicine will focus on the head; when you have foot pains, then Western medicine will be used to examine the foot. Traditional Chinese Medicine links humans with the universe – the 'oneness of universe and our human body'. Chinese medicine looks at the whole person, and is good for preventive health care and chronic illness.

In Western biomedical discourse, the focus is individualistic and on organ systems and components of the body. Typically, disease is viewed as 'impairment in the functioning of any single component, or of the relationship between [the] components that make up the individual' (Curtis & Taket 1996:26). Conversely, as we will see throughout this book, the rationale of Traditional Chinese Medicine focuses on the close relationship between an individual and the universe or environment; in *Nei Jing*, for instance, the importance of understanding the whole social and natural environment for treating a patient is emphasised.

As a result of political change, the holistic approach to health was reinvigorated in mid-twentieth century China. People recognised the importance of the unity of the parts and the whole (both relating to the body and in general terms) which, although appearing to oppose one another, at the same time constitute a homogenous entity. The parts and whole are related and one cannot exist without another; if there are no parts, there is also no whole. Mencius (trans. Dobson 1963:144) spoke of the importance of caring for the parts within the whole:

A man cares about all parts of his body without discrimination, and so he nurtures all parts equally. There is not a square inch of skin that he does not care about, and so he tends all his skin equally... A doctor who treats one finger and neglects the back and shoulder would be a very befuddled physician.

Cai Jingfeng (蔡景峰), a modern Professor in the history of Chinese medicine with training in both Western and Traditional Chinese Medicine, commented that for Western medicine, the treatment target is specifically the disease and the diseased organ, while in Chinese medicine, the target is the whole patient, together with the patient's physiological function which is believed to be off-balance (Pearce 2001).

Natural means of restoring energy

A 50-year-old man in Armidale (originally from Taiwan) spoke of the 'natural' way of Traditional Chinese Medicine:

Traditional Chinese Medicine is more 'natural' than Western medicine, without side effects... This helps to recover 'energy' in our bodies.

He articulated three ideas regarding Traditional Chinese Medicine: that it is natural, that is less prone to side-effects; and that it has an energy-boosting capacity. In Traditional Chinese Medicine, body and nature are considered together. In *Nei Jing*, the emphasis is on adhering to nature in order to maintain a healthy balance, with chapter twenty-five delineating 'the principle of nature in treatment'.

This man also viewed Traditional Chinese Medicine as having fewer side effects. However, a survey conducted in 1996 by Australian researchers (Bensoussan, Myers & Carlton 2000) on the side-effects of herbs and acupuncture indicates that the use of herbal medicine is not problem-free. Researchers in that study identified problems associated with Traditional Chinese Medicine that included allergic reactions, interactions with prescription drugs, toxic impurities, and the improper mixing of herbs. Other researchers have also raised concerns about the side-effects of Traditional Chinese Medicine (see Siegel 1979; Lee 1980; Ng, Chan & Yu 1991; Gorey, Wahlqvist & Boyce 1992; Vanherweghem, Depierreux & Tielemans 1993).

'Energy' has profound significance in Traditional Chinese Medicine, and the loss of vital energy is a sign of bodily imbalance. Energy embraces everything; it is a unifying force that binds everything together – our body system and our way of living. The whole universe is dependent on this energy or *qi*, which contributes to the brightness of the stars, the formation of weather, the causation of the seasons, and the supports for man's survival (Hammer 1990).

Energy ensures the health of a person, as suggested by a 30-year-old Western man, a martial arts teacher living in Brisbane:

> Energy is a combination of breath, blood circulation, and *qi* energy. So whenever you are sick, a channel gets blocked, like the garden hose that has been bent. So the Chinese therapy – be it massage or acupuncture, Qi Gong or Tai Chi – works on getting the *qi* to go through the channel where the blockage is.

This man also spoke of two positive uses of *qi*: for health, such as in breathing and physical exercises; and for defence, to condition one's body and to absorb impact. He also spoke of the negative use of *qi* in an attack, such as by using *qi* to punch someone with such force as to cause damage to internal organs.

A comprehensive explanation of the meaning of *qi* energy can be found in *Nei Jing* (*Spiritual Pivot*, chapter 54:718), which defines the levels of energy and associated activities appropriate for various life stages from 10 to 100 years of age. The following table is constructed according to that text:

Age	Energy level	Motor activity
10	unimpeded	running
20	prosperous	walking fast
30	reduced	walk slowing
40	(not specified)	sitting
50	declining of liver energy	(not specified)
60	declining of heat energy	lying down
70	weakening of spleen energy	(not specified)
80	declining of lung energy	out of order
90	withering of kidney energy	not functioning
100	all empty with no spirit	may die at any time

'Energy' at various ages of life.

(*Spiritual Pivot*, chapter 54:718)

Source of beliefs

Participants drew their bases for comparing Traditional Chinese Medicine and Western medicine from two sources – documentary evidence and personal experience.

A characteristic of recent Western culture is the use of scientific reasoning, which is manifested by people using logical methods and having an attitude of inquiry and an analytic spirit. Some participants' underlying beliefs were strongly influenced by this 'enlightenment' mode of thinking.

Scientific medical discourses

In Western medical discourse, the body is often viewed through the metaphor of a machine that can be repaired. The belief is that in order to know the function of a part, such as an organ, it needs to be taken apart, hence the need to dissect corpses. Benjamin Hobson recognised this in 1875 in his *Summary of Western Medicine* (Unschuld 1985), when he noted the Chinese doctors' lack of experience in dissection and lack of knowledge concerning the organs and the origins of illness. In this regard, Traditional Chinese Medicine was considered unsophisticated. However, Sivin (2003) argues that the lack of details about anatomy and physiology in Traditional Chinese Medicine was not a handicap in itself; in Europe, anatomical knowledge only began to be used in health care in the early nineteenth century. Surgery based on reliable anatomical information was not available in the United States until around 1920.

The advantages of Western medicine for surgical procedures were expressed by an 80-year-old man in Brisbane (originally from Hong Kong), who believed that both medical models had their place, depending on the severity of the problem:

> I believe Traditional Chinese Medicine is good for minor problems. However, for major problems that require operations you have to rely on Western medicine for surgery.

A preference for Western medicine voiced by a 35-year-old woman in Sydney (originally from Hong Kong) was ostensibly based on scientific reasoning, as reflected by the participant's criteria of evaluation: evidence with supporting theory, objectivity, clear explanations. She felt it was important to have an understanding of the effects of medicine on the body, and that such a scientific approach would also provide credibility to a practitioner of Traditional Chinese Medicine:

> Western medicine is evidence-based; you know the theory behind it. For example, taking antibiotics too long may cause stomach upset because it kills the *E. coli* in the intestine. There is no such writing in Traditional Chinese Medicine. To a certain extent I do believe in Traditional Chinese Medicine, if the doctor is objective and backed up by theory – one who is clear in whatever he or she does and can explain everything.

A 69-year-old man in Brisbane (originally from Papua New Guinea) expressed the opinion that medicine needs to be tested, regardless of its source:

> Medicine is taken for a cure, whether it is Traditional Chinese Medicine or Western medicine. If it has the effect of healing, then it should be taken, regardless of whether it is Traditional Chinese Medicine or Western. If it produces the effects that it should, take it. Yes, but it has to be scientifically tested.

A 77-year-old man in Sydney (originally from Mainland China) also preferred Traditional Chinese Medicine to be backed by scientific analysis.

From his personal experience in treating tinea (the so-called 'Hong Kong foot'), he preferred Western medicine for particular situations. He suggests combining Western medicine and Traditional Chinese Medicine to treat chronic illness:

> I cannot believe in Traditional Chinese Medicine that has no proper analysis. For example, I had fungus on my toes, called by the Chinese 'Hong Kong foot' (香港腳), which could not be treated by Traditional Chinese Medicine. I had to rely on Western medicine for treatment. For chronic illness, three methods should be combined: first, Western diagnosis through pathological analysis; second, the use of good Traditional Chinese Medicine doctors; third, the use of food therapy.

In Brisbane, the middle-aged group (originally from Taiwan) expresses a dependency on Western medicine by saying:

> In life we cannot abandon Western medicine, but we can go without Traditional Chinese Medicine.

They noted that in Taiwan, Traditional Chinese Medicine and Western medicine are combined, but many people place greater trust in Western medicine. One striking cultural difference they noted between the practice of Western medicine in Australia and in Taiwan was that doctors in Australia resisted prescribing medications for minor illnesses. The general advice they gave is to 'have a good rest and plenty of water'. By contrast, doctors in Taiwan tended to rely more heavily on giving injections.

This group largely equated Traditional Chinese Medicine with 'food therapy', used for therapeutic purposes, for invigorating health, and as an ordinary health supplement. They insisted that Traditional Chinese Medicine needs more scientific evidence, testing, and clinical trials.

They also noted a lack of good textbooks in Traditional Chinese Medicine. Traditional Chinese Medicine is not standardised and there appear to be mysterious principles that are difficult for lay people to grasp, such as the conceptual division of body types and foods into 'hot and cold'. They blamed this lack of standardised terms on historical circumstances:

> In the ancient times, the ancestors did not have the language to describe. They could only use the simplest terms and metaphors to describe some discomfort.

Western medicine was felt to provide more direction and proof; tests can be performed to support a diagnosis, and acute or serious bodily malfunctions can generally be detected and fixed quickly. Some Traditional Chinese Medicines were considered very good, but unrefined.

Personal experience

Although many participants endorsed the need for 'scientific evidence' in the use of any medicine, some participants clung to their beliefs based on personal experience. This approach constitutes empirical rather than scientific evidence, especially when they view their experience as trustworthy and obtaining the desired effect (Blair 1995). In pre-modern times, the use of Traditional Chinese Medicine was based on experience and belief (Unschuld 1985).

Personal experiences were generally the main reason that participants believed in Traditional Chinese Medicine. A 27-year-old woman (born in Hong Kong but now living in Sydney) said that Traditional Chinese Medicine could minimise the need for high dosages and the side effects of Western medicine:

> Western medicine is very good at doing surgery, but when it comes to diagnosing skin disorders and nose allergies, I find Traditional Chinese Medicine better. I find the more Western medicine antibiotics you take, the higher the dose you will need. Chinese medicine, on the other hand, has fewer side effects which even a weak body can tolerate.

This woman in Sydney had complaints of various kinds; on the advice of her mother she decided to try Traditional Chinese Medicine. She realised her body had become weak under the influence of too many fried and cold foods. She used to have two to three bars of chocolate and sometimes 250 g of lollies per day. Moreover, she said five out of ten foods in the Chinese vegetarian restaurant were sweet things like water-chestnut and tofu puddings, and she would have them all. She said 'my allergy is mainly from inside my body'. She decided to abstain from fried, sweet and cold foods, and considered Traditional Chinese Medicine as part of her food supplements.

This 45-year-old man in Armidale (originally from Beijing, Mainland China) found from personal experience that he admired the qualities of Traditional Chinese Medicine doctors:

> My belief in Traditional Chinese Medicine depends on whether Traditional Chinese Medicine doctors are of top quality or not. Many people go to see top quality doctors, who are mostly older.

This man associated 'top quality' doctors with high status and considered them to be famous doctors who are sought after and considered above average. In China, it is common to line up to see famous doctors, based on word of mouth. He also equated age with experience.

A 48-year-old woman in Sydney (originally from Hong Kong) preferred to use Traditional Chinese Medicine to keep her energy going in order to cope with her busy life. She could afford even fairly expensive Traditional Chinese Medicine, which she believed kept her healthy and gave her the drive to succeed:

> I continue to boil these medicines to keep my health, for I know that without good health I cannot work. Some time ago I was rather weak and I prepared Traditional Chinese Medicine frequently. I did not rest from work, but kept on eating Chinese Medicine. When I had money I bought the medicine. I boiled lots of Chinese medicine to keep me healthy.

This woman would work and work until she could not go on, from the time she was a child. She neglected her health and ate an unbalanced diet:

> I had one salted egg for two meals, together with boiled white rice. I had that for three years, because I wanted to save money; one salted egg cost 25 cents ($Hong Kong) and I had to pay rent. I did not care if it was nice to eat or not.

Money meant security and happiness to her. She thought that with money she could buy everything; she said she felt happy when 'I press the button on the calculator to see how much money I have, and the dollars goes up'. When her health suffered, she believed Traditional Chinese Medicine would help her regain her health.

Another Hong Kong experience was shared by a woman living in Armidale. She perceived Traditional Chinese Medicine as a supplement largely because of her mother's influence. This participant used Western medicine more than Traditional Chinese Medicine. While still in Hong Kong, she would sometimes try Chinese herbs before consulting a Western doctor. One time she took her child with a rash to a Western hospital in Hong Kong. The doctor, who knew her well, said:

> Have you given the child that Chinese skin-cream? What about that Chinese cough syrup and the pill for safeguarding babies? I think they did not work, and that is why you are here today.

Though she was less keen on using Traditional Chinese Medicine for her children, she learnt a lot from her mother, who used to cook for doctors in a Hong Kong hospital. Her mother related well to the doctors; when the doctors did not feel well, they would say to her mother, 'Sister, we should try your Chinese herbal tea'. Then her mother would recommend some popular Traditional Chinese Medicine.

For a 45-year-old man in Sydney (originally from Hong Kong), his experience of Traditional Chinese Medicine came from word-of-mouth recommendations and convenience:

> I used to work in Central (Hong Kong), where I could buy ready-made Chinese Medicine drinks… Many people went there. I drank it because I heard other people saying that herbal teas were good.

In the main administrative centre in Hong Kong, where this man worked, many shops offer Traditional Chinese Medicine herbal teas for people in a hurry. Again, popularity of a product or a service was equated with good quality and word-of-mouth recommendations were trusted.

Transmission of Traditional Chinese Medicine knowledge

Passing on knowledge of Traditional Chinese Medicine is fundamental for the continuity and survival of Traditional Chinese Medicine. Participants were concerned that knowledge about Traditional Chinese Medicine is not freely available, perhaps even withheld.

This is large attributable to the teaching tradition for Traditional Chinese Medicine, which is based on individual experience and oral transmission. This phenomenon is prevalent in the villages and rural areas and in traditional family practices, in which the 'folk medicine' or indigenous medical ways have been handed down from generation to generation. Traditionally, transmission of Traditional Chinese Medicine knowledge has been from father to son or from master to apprentice (Zhang & Rose 1999), usually through oral accounts with some complementary written texts (Holbrook 1977).

Oral tradition

A 77-year-old man in Sydney (originally from Mainland China) pointed out that reliance on memory and oral traditions has limited the transmission of 'folk medicine' or traditional family practices. Knowledge is acquired through experience without documentation or consistent standards:

Much knowledge of Traditional Chinese Medicine was handed down from generation to generation, and some is difficult to understand. The difficulty of passing the knowledge on is compounded by the fact that much knowledge of Traditional Chinese Medicine depends on memory.

These constraints on access to knowledge about Traditional Chinese Medicine lead to people having limited exposure to and reservations about traditional practices, and thus developing a preference for Western medicine, as indicated by a 27-year-old woman in Sydney (originally from Hong Kong):

> I think it is difficult to carry the torch of Traditional Chinese Medicine because of the restrained manner towards passing knowledge of Traditional Chinese Medicine on. Western medicine is more advanced. People often learn from their parents.

Knowledge within the family

A 58-year-old woman in Sydney (originally from Mainland China) said that action speaks louder than words, and that the practice of Traditional Chinese Medicine was best taught in the family by preparing and performing it in front of one's children. She was confident that her children's generation will pass on Traditional Chinese Medicine knowledge in a similar manner. She set a fine example of sharing knowledge of Traditional Chinese Medicine in her family.

On the other hand, a 35-year-old woman in Sydney (originally from Hong Kong) suggested that if parents did not believe in or use Traditional Chinese Medicine, the next generation would be unlikely to learn about it. Besides, the next generation has the choice of Western medicine. She did not see herself as traditional, believed in Western medicine, and commented that antibiotics could replace many Traditional Chinese Medicine remedies.

She mentioned that her family had knowledge of many secret formulas, yet her father did not pass on Traditional Chinese Medicine wisdom to her on the grounds that she would not understand it. Moreover:

> In passing on knowledge of Traditional Chinese Medicine, if there are ten types of Traditional Chinese Medicine knowledge, one will be kept behind. Therefore, one can only pass on nine types of Traditional Chinese Medicine knowledge to others. This is particularly true due to people's 'selfish nature'.

The unwillingness of this woman's father to pass Traditional Chinese Medicine knowledge on to her can perhaps be explained by the traditional Chinese family practice of passing knowledge down from father to sons, not to daughters. Secret formulas become 'family treasures' and thus 'jealously guarded secrets' (Zhang & Rose 1999). Giving away Traditional Chinese Medicine knowledge is equated with giving away your treasury. Girls will marry and give their knowledge to another family. Because of this closed system of transmission, traditional knowledge is easily lost.

Teachers withhold knowledge for a reason

However, a 50-year-old man in Armidale (originally from Taiwan) shared his concerns that a person knowledgeable in Traditional Chinese Medicine might not pass all that knowledge on to next generation in fear that the follower could usurp the teacher. The three-generation attitude, a popular saying among the Chinese, would further restrict the successful transmission of Traditional Chinese Medicine knowledge through the generations:

> During the course of passing on Traditional Chinese Medicine knowledge, the first generation would glorify and create, the next generation would maintain the knowledge, and the third generation would show no interest... This is due to the 'falling human nature'. There is a saying 'teaching followers the full knowledge would end up with no masters' (教識徒弟沒師父).

'Teaching followers the full knowledge would end up with no masters' implies that students have an ungrateful attitude and will not defer to their teachers. This saying also projects the inner insecurity of teachers and mistrust between teachers and students. These reservations have their roots in traditional Chinese culture (Wai 1995). In agricultural societies, people tend to be more reserved because of their simple lifestyle. This reserved manner promotes social solidarity and, at the same time, self-centredness.

The difficulty in passing on Traditional Chinese Medicine knowledge is compounded by assumptions that new generations do not want to work as hard as prior generations, reflected in the Chinese saying that 'from the father's generation cannot pass through three generations'. This participant attributed this failure to human weakness. Some people prefer to simply accept existing knowledge rather than taking risks to be creative and make new breakthroughs.

A 45-year-old man in Sydney (originally from Hong Kong) commented that teachers should hold the dominant role and students should not surpass teachers, because students would not have the experience and practice that the teachers had:

> I do not think that there is a problem of passing on knowledge of Traditional Chinese Medicine. I think students should not surpass their teachers. For example, I teach you something, at least I learnt it first. Even though I teach you all that I know, what you learn is only the beginning. Some knowledge needs experience and practice, and hard work in order to understand.

In traditional Chinese society, teachers have high status and are much honoured, second only in position to one's parents. This participant suggested, therefore, that students should be humble in learning.

Teaching as a virtue

Other participants held positive views about transmitting knowledge of Traditional Chinese Medicine fully. A 62-year-old male practitioner of Traditional Chinese Medicine in Sydney (originally from Mainland China), said he had no reservations about teaching:

> If I know, I would teach my students; if I teach, I would teach without reservations. If people really want to serve people, and consider humanity as their great aim, they would show no reservation in teaching.

This Traditional Chinese Medicine practitioner was a firm believer in Tao, and said it was his primary aim to serve his fellow men based on the humanistic teachings of Taoism. He said those who are committed to serve would teach people Traditional Chinese Medicine, regardless of whether they were rich or poor, as long as they were keen to learn.

Another enthusiastic teacher was a 30-year-old Australian man who had been teaching Martial Arts and Traditional Chinese Medicine for fifteen years to disciples in Brisbane:

> For me, being a good teacher means I hope my students can be better than me. That means I have done a good job. I know the Chinese way is not to give the students everything; others may hold something as reserve to let the students find out for themselves what is more important and more useful to them.

After twelve years with his own instructor, who had returned to Taiwan, this Western man was aware of the Chinese practice of reservation in teaching. His instructor had not told him much directly. The Western man just realised that his instructor wanted him to work things out for himself. The Western participant, however, said he was open with his knowledge and would be proud of his students should they surpass him.

Also in Brisbane, a 30-year-old woman (originally from Papua New Guinea) used the metaphor of 'growing a pie' in reference to passing on knowledge of Traditional Chinese Medicine. The implication was that knowledge is cumulative:

> I think passing on knowledge of Traditional Chinese Medicine is like growing a pie, not reducing it. To me, knowledge is something that grows and grows. When you reduce the pie, knowledge suffers. Someone who is in power, someone who is insecure, in control, will never cause things to grow.

Helping others means helping oneself, as recognised in the *Analects* (Book 6, chapter 28:2): 'Now the man of perfect virtue, wishing to be established himself, seeks also to establish others; wishing to enlarge himself, he seeks to enlarge others'. In contrast, the fear of passing knowledge on implies a lack of trust and insecurity.

Similarly, the view of a 27-year-old man in Brisbane (originally from Vietnam) reflected the traditional Confucian teaching of adhering to the social role of the individual:

> It is a pity that some Traditional Chinese Medicine doctors are selfish and will not pass their full knowledge on. A master should do the duty of a master, and a student should have the duty of a student. The master has a duty to teach, and a student should try one's best to learn. The right moral concept should be like that.

He perceived that practitioners who withhold knowledge are acting incompatibly with the moral teaching of Confucius that each of us should carry out our duty as best we can. Regarding teaching, Confucius generally advocated equal opportunity for all students (學不厭教不倦); however, on the individual level, he was keen to pass on his knowledge to those students who were eager and aware.

Attitude of the learner

Passing on knowledge of Traditional Chinese Medicine also depends on the attitude of the learners as well as that of the teachers or parents:

> When teaching Traditional Chinese Medicine in the traditional Chinese way, teachers used to consider the followers' character – whether they showed filial piety, and would not cause trouble. Learning depends on 'awareness'. This is easier said than done... People in the past believed, 'When Heaven is about to confer a great office on any man, it first exercises his mind with suffering, and his sinews and bones with toil'. People in the past could tolerate hardship, but who can do this in this modern world?

In expressing this view, a 62-year-old man in Sydney (originally from Mainland China) referred to the importance of the relationship between instructors and followers as well as the qualities of the individual followers. Encounters between teacher and follower are considered *yuan* (緣), which generally refers to the luck of meeting, the predestined lot, and the affinity that binds people together. In the traditional Chinese way, instructors would pass on knowledge of Traditional Chinese Medicine if the followers showed 'filial piety'. In the case of followers showing 'filial piety' towards their instructors, their attitudes should embrace loyalty, respect and obedience.

As for individual qualities, this participant believed that 'awareness' was needed in order to understand knowledge passed on by instructors. Not all students possess this great gift whereby, as the Chinese saying records, 'once one learns the first word, one can be aware of the rest' (話頭醒尾). Confucius also spoke of this attitude towards learning and the awareness of the student (*Analects*, Book 7, chapter 8). Regarding learning, a student should show eagerness and readiness. In addition, a student should have awareness, that is, the ability to see through things. Otherwise, a student was not qualified to be his student. This attitude towards learning is 'easier said than done' – it is easier to say than to do, and the emphasis is on action. Action was basic in Confucius's teachings. Confucius defined virtues such as filial piety, humanness and loyalty in terms of human relationships, to be expressed through daily actions.

This 62-year-old man in Sydney also noted that while people in the past were willing to study hard to master Traditional Chinese Medicine, this is not the case in the modern world. When he spoke of virtuous and learned people tending to undergo hardships before they gained recognition, he was referring to the teachings of Mencius.

Reflections

This chapter uncovers people's beliefs about the roles and functions of Traditional Chinese Medicine relative to Western medicine, sources of authority for each of the medical models, and the transmission of Traditional Chinese Medicine knowledge.

The participants' responses concerning the relative positioning of Traditional Chinese Medicine and Western medicine suggested three main considerations. Firstly, the two medical models enrich each other and each has a role to play. Western medicine was seen to excel in surgery, offering quick relief and lowering temperature efficiently; the taste and colour of modern medicines were also more appealing to the younger-aged group participants from Hong Kong. Traditional Chinese Medicine, on the other hand, was believed to work well for chronic illnesses and to have fewer side effects. Secondly, Western medicine was seen to focus on the discrete organs and disease, whereas Traditional Chinese Medicine Traditional emphasises the whole person as well as his or her environment. Thirdly, Traditional Chinese Medicine was considered a more natural means of restoring 'energy'.

Two areas of interest were identified in the participants' underlying beliefs about the authority of each of the medical models, regarding scientific evidence and personal experience. Participants argued that scientific advancement in Traditional Chinese Medicine was lacking. This belief was particularly supported by the group of middle-aged participants from Taiwan who perceived Traditional Chinese Medicine to be inseparable from 'food therapy'. Participants' experiences of using Traditional Chinese Medicine influenced their trust in Traditional Chinese Medicine, and this seemed to be far more important than scientific proof in influencing their decisions to use Traditional Chinese Medicine.

Participants expressed concerns about how knowledge of Traditional Chinese Medicine is passed on. Reasons which account for the withholding of knowledge were given as the reserved nature of Chinese culture, family traditions, human selfishness, personal insecurity, mistrust between instructors and followers, and reliance on memory and oral traditions.

An important point is that transmission of Traditional Chinese Medicine knowledge by instructors depends on the individual qualities of students, namely whether they show filial piety to instructors, have an awareness of Traditional Chinese Medicine, and display a willingness to work hard. Traditionally, students are not supposed to surpass teachers in the sense that, as learners, they lack the experience of their instructors. Therefore, students should be humble and instructors and students should play their roles accordingly.

Another issue was the traditional role of families in the transmission of Traditional Chinese Medicine knowledge. Children learn Traditional Chinese Medicine from seeing and using Traditional Chinese Medicine as practiced by their parents. The advantage of passing on knowledge was described by the metaphor of 'growing a pie' – knowledge is cumulative, and so it should help to increase the pie, thus helping the body of knowledge to grow.

The vital dimension of the philosophical aspect of Traditional Chinese Medicine, in terms of the balancing effect of Traditional Chinese Medicine in restoring harmony in life, is explored next. This 'harmony' provides a pervasive guiding principle in health, whether the balancing relates to the human being in the environment, emotional wellbeing, or foods. The underlying principle of harmony in the philosophy of living is the focus of the following chapter.

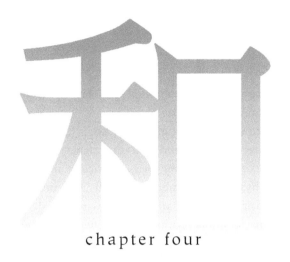

chapter four

Balance and Harmony

(Pronounced as *huo*, which refers to 'harmony', recognising differences
and co-existence)

All things nurture together without harming each other.
Each pursues its own way without opposing each other.

The Doctrine of the Mean, chapter 30 (my translation)

Introduction

The concepts of balance and harmony have profound implications in
Traditional Chinese Medicine as in Chinese culture. According to the
medical theory of Traditional Chinese Medicine, *yin* and *yang* harmony is
necessary for good health; either form in excess is believed to cause disharmony
and is a prelude to illness. Metaphors such as wind and heat, from outside our
bodies to the emotions inside, are perceived as contributing factors in the
initiation of various types of illness. This concept is based on the understanding

of the unity or harmonious relationship between the microcosm of humans and the macrocosm of the universe.

Yin and yang embrace diverse meanings. Sivin (2003) points out that they belong to everyday language and that they have specialised meanings in learned discourse. Yin and yang are significant in Traditional Chinese Medicine, as physical and mental health are inseparable from this complementary pair. Once the yin and yang are out of balance, disease is inevitable. This harmonious relationship is reflected in the Tao. To live in balance, without going to extremes, is one of the highest ideals of Taoist philosophy. Tao Te Ching (chapter 9, trans. Lau 1963) has this to say on not going to extremes:

> Rather than fill it to the brim by keeping it upright, better to have stopped in time.
> Hammer it to the point, and the sharpness cannot be preserved forever.
> There may be gold and jade to fill a hall, but there is none who can keep them.

Balance and avoiding extremes was recommended as a means of maintaining health by the Tang Dynasty physician, Sun Si-miao (581–682 CE), in his 'doing less' guide:

> One who knows how to conserve one's life is one who thinks less, worries less, has less desire, is less active, talks less, is less upset, has less joy, has less anger, and does less wrong.

> (Quoted in Lin & Flaws 1991:17)

In Sun's view, harmony embraces conserving one's mental and spiritual energy and avoiding excess. Doing less is a typical Taoist view of 'non-intervention' and of not going to extremes. Sun was a Tao follower, like many physicians who practiced Traditional Chinese Medicine in those days. Lin and Flaws (1991) argued that 'doing less' seems impossible in modern times because of our links to the material world. However, the wisdom of 'less', that is, not going to extremes, is an important element underlying the philosophy of Traditional Chinese Medicine.

The balance of yin and yang is 'a metaphor for sustaining adaptability and equilibrium' (Beinfield & Korngold 1991:50). According to this view, balance is characterised by flexibility, diversity, moderation, and the balance of one's rhythms and needs. Tao suggests this balance is the balance between the individual and the environment. The concepts of *yin* and *yang* balance are articulated in *Nei Jing*:

> The *yin* and *yang* within a human body must always be kept in balance. The over-abundance of *yin* will cause *yang* diseases and the over-abundance of *yang* will cause *yin* disease.

(Plain Questions chapter 5:33)

Imbalance in Hammer's (1990:96–98) opinion means the extremes of normal function. He gives an example of hallucinations as a sign of extremes, of lacking strong and controlled boundaries. Extremes are sometimes needed to effect change or restore imbalance, but as a way of life they are considered destructive. Furthermore, excess or deficiency of *yin* and *yang* is interpreted as disharmony in the context from which it arises, either constitutional or from life experience. According to Hammer's view, no one is totally 'in balance'.

From the medical point of view, *yin* and *yang* provide insights for diagnosis, treatment and pathology in Traditional Chinese Medicine. *Nei Jing* (*Plain Questions*, chapter 5:42) records the diagnosis of *yin* and *yang*, which is determined by observing the complexion and pulse of patients. Red complexion indicates *yang*, white complexion indicates *yin*; floating pulse is *yang*, and deep pulse is *yin*. For treating disease, the variation in *yin* and *yang* provides the guiding principle (*Nei Jing*, *Plain Questions*, chapter 5). The holistic approach of embracing the physical and mental aspects of patients in order to restore health fully is suggested: 'In treating, one can always keep the orderliness by inspecting the breath and the mental attitude of the patient' (*Nei Jing*, *Plain Questions*, chapter 80:484).

Regarding the relationship of *yin* and *yang* to pathology, the term 'lucid energy' is used to refer to *yang* energy, and 'turbid energy' refers to *yin* energy. In adverse health conditions, the *yang* energy (heavenly energy) descends, while *yin* energy (earthly energy) ascends. This formulation of 'heat–evil' attributes pathological change to an imbalance between these two energies in the form of a 'disturbance above' (*Nei Jing*, *Plain Questions*, chapter 5:3). Any imbalance is believed to cause a disturbance in the natural flow of energy such that, eventually, *qi* – the vital energy – is blocked, resulting in illness. Traditional Chinese Medicine uses various methods to restore the *yin* and *yang* balance.

The meanings that the participants ascribed to *yin* and *yang* revealed four aspects of interest: the concept of the *yin* and *yang* balance, balance in foods, disease as caused by imbalance, and harmony in living. These aspects provide insights into the dynamic human and cosmic phenomena stemming from *yin* and *yang*. These concepts suggest complementarities and co–existence, and they inject meaning into Traditional Chinese Medicine.

Balance through yin and yang

A 39-year-old man in Armidale (originally from Shanghai, Mainland China), expressed the concept of *yin* and *yang* in this way:

> There are three main concepts of *yin* and *yang*: of one into two, of complementing each other, and of being dynamic and changing. Imbalance of either side may cause illness.

In this quote are framed the concepts of co–existence, constant change, transformation and dynamism.

Another view of *yin* and *yang* was expressed by a 50-year-old man in Armidale (originally from Taiwan):

> Everyone has both *yin* and *yang*. In Traditional Chinese Medicine, medicine is used for *yin* or *yang* purposes. For example, a male may need *yin* or *yang* medicine depending on his condition. A man needs *yin* and *yang* balance.

Excessive *yang* contributes to heat syndromes; excessive *yin* produces cold syndromes; deficient *yang* leads to hyperactivity of *yin* and cold syndromes of a deficient type; and deficient *yin* leads to heat syndromes of a weak type (Xu 2001). Not surprisingly then, Traditional Chinese Medicine drugs are divided according to *yin* and *yang* principles. The four types of drugs are cold, hot, warm, and cool, which are classified according to their pharmacological features. The *yin* drugs are the cold and cool ones; and the *yang* types are hot and warm types. A person may need both types of Traditional Chinese Medicine. *Yin* and *yang* Traditional Chinese Medicines are chosen firstly on the basis of the causes of illness, and secondly to address the imbalance of *yin* and *yang*.

Balance with the environment

A 32-year-old woman in Brisbane (originally from Papua New Guinea) expressed this view about the need for individuals to be in balance with their environment:

I think of *yin* and *yang* as balancing in your life like harmony, with yourself, with your environment, and with everything.

Another perspective is provided by a 62-year-old man in Sydney (originally from See Yup, Mainland China), who reflects on the lack of balance inherent in modern lifestyles:

From the view of Traditional Chinese Medicine, it is critical to see why people's *yin* and *yang* is not balanced. Some people have late nights, their health is subjected to stress, and the external evils would attack their bodies, resulting in *yin* and *yang* imbalance.

From this quote emerges two themes relating to Traditional Chinese Medicine ideas about causes of disease in an unbalance body – emotional 'stress', and 'external evils' (discussed later in this chapter). 'Stress' is considered the worst form of harm to health, because it combines all the negative energies that have detrimental impacts on the immune system (Reid 1996:54). Similarly, evidence from Western medical research also indicates stress can have a negative impact on our bodies by causing physiological changes in hormones, nervous system, blood pressure and immune system (Shilling 1993:116). Another explanation of the hazard of any emotional disturbances, such as anger, joy, excessive sorrow, fear, fright, and worry, is that it may affect the natural flow of the vital energy, *qi* (Lin & Flaws 1991:11).

Balancing emotions

A 48-year-old woman in Sydney (originally from Hong Kong) articulates the balance of *yin* and *yang* in emotions as follows:

I think of *yin* and *yang* balance in terms of people's emotions, which cause fluctuations in moods and affect people's health.

In Traditional Chinese Medicine, good emotional health is a requisite for healthy living. Emotions are perceived as 'energy–in–motion'; when too intense, emotions can upset the harmony of the bodily systems (Reid 1996:53). Traditional Chinese Medicine identifies 'Seven Emotions' that affect health – joy, anger, anxiety, worry, grief, fear, and fright. *Nei Jing* (*Plain Questions*, chapter 19) refers to 'Five Emotions': 'over-joy may hurt the heart', 'anger hurts the liver', 'anxiety hurts the spleen', 'terror hurts the kidney', and 'melancholy hurts the lung.' These emotional factors are the main causes for internal disease according to Traditional Chinese Medicine. On the other hand, 'high' human emotions such as love, compassion, and devotion are seen to have a positive effect on health.

I Ching also illustrates the link between negative emotions and physical ill health. In the hexagram that illuminates 'breakthrough' ☰, *I Ching* states that, 'There is no skin on his thighs and walking becomes hard' (Baynes 1965:169). This brings to mind the image of a person whose thighs had previously been strong, but who had been weakened by emotional disturbance. However, on other occasions, emotional upset may result in positive outcomes. The symbolic expression of six lines at the top of the *I Ching* hexagram ☷ representing 'gathering together' argues that 'lamenting and sighing, flood of tears' is considered positive and conducive to positive outcomes (Baynes 1965:177). Initially, one is upset because one's good intention to form an alliance with another person is misunderstood. Eventually, the other person understands and the alliance is established or the grief is resolved.

Balance in food

Food is described as being the essence of life in *Nei Jing*:

> Man takes in food of five tastes and absorbs its essence to nourish the body. The essence of life depends on the healthy energy, and the shaping up of the physique depends on the food (taste). The food, when being digested and transformed, turns into the essence of life which can finally substantialise the physique.
>
> (*Plain Questions*, chapter 5:32)

It was recommended that a diet should include all five tastes – sweet, bitter, acrid (hot and strong favour), sour and salty, to build the body and maintain balance.

In contemporary Western settings, a balanced diet is considered in terms of the nutritional properties of foods in the five food groups (Smith, Kellett & Schmerlaib 1998:5).

In Traditional Chinese Medicine, however, foods are divided according to *yin* and *yang* properties attributed to them, which are considered to be the primary influence on our physical, emotional, and spiritual health. Eating too much or too little of either may cause imbalance. Generally speaking, foods within the *yin* spectrum include vegetables, fruits, sweetened foods, soft drinks, tea and coffee. *Yang* foods include most meats, poultry and eggs. Foods with a balance of *yin* and *yang* include grains, seeds and beans. Generally, the ancient doctor Sun Si-miao recommended these latter foods as well as vegetables and fruits whose flavours are naturally light and harmonious for a balanced diet (cited in Sun 1988). But Sun Si-miao did not exclude meat from a healthy diet, as he went on to say, 'Eat those fish, meat and fruit which boost people's health' (Sun Si-miao, quoted in Flaws 1994:22).

The *yin* in Traditional Chinese Medicine is considered to nourish and build women's blood, while the *yang* Traditional Chinese Medicine is suitable for men's vital energy, as suggested by this 56-year-old woman in Armidale (originally from Hong Kong):

> Traditional Chinese Medicine is divided into *yin* and *yang*. *Dong quan* is *yin* that is good for females. *Redmedler berry* is *yang* and is good for males.

(Note that *redmedler berry* is commonly used for both males and females. These small red seeds are highly nutritious and believed to be beneficial for the eyes and building blood. They go well with *yang* medicine and *yang* meats for strengthening the bodies of both males and females.)

Another belief is that the type of cooking also affect the qualities of foods. Adding more heat, such as by deep-frying or roasting, would increase the *yang* qualities of foods. Cooking by steaming (and more recently by microwave) is *yin*. Stir-frying over gas is considered a balanced approach.

In the view of a 39-year-old woman in Armidale (originally from New Zealand), a variety of types and colours of food were important for balancing her body. Her only contact with Traditional Chinese Medicine had been through foods that she was particularly interested in. Therefore, she viewed *yin* and *yang* as harmonising one's daily living through food and balanced relationships with the environment:

> *Yin* and *yang* refers to the balance of positive and negative food and energy, energy from the sun, garden, walking around in bare feet. This is how I balance myself.

The interdependence of humankind with heaven and earth is echoed in *Nei Jing (Plain Questions*, chapter 5), where three types of energies are identified: the *yang* energy of heaven that nourishes one's head; the *yin* energy of earth that nourishes one's feet, and in the middle one can use foods to regulate one's body.

Seasonal considerations

A 39-year-old man in Armidale (originally from Shanghai, Mainland China) points out how food practices are adjusted according to the seasons:

> In winter, I eat lamb by preparing it with red dates, which is a good *yang* food to keep me warm. Summer is a good time for regulating *yin*, and I should take *yin* food instead.

Nutritious foods in winter are congruent with the Traditional Chinese Medicine principle that winter is the ideal time for supplements and nourishment. There are two ways of nourishing our bodies: medicines and food. The latter is considered preferable: 'Food supplements are better than medicine supplements' (Yiu 1984:82). It is generally believed that eating well in winter can prevent disease. Lamb is *yang* food, a warm food, which is good for winter. The Chinese dried red dates are believed to be good for blood building. Summer, on the other hand, is a time for the growth of *yin*, and lighter foods are recommended.

According to Traditional Chinese Medicine, the consumption of foods should be adjusted in accordance with the four seasons and the five tastes as discussed in chapters two and three of *Nei Jing*. In this way, disease is prevented by following nature. Spring belongs to the growth of *yang*; the liver is strengthened at this stage. Gentle warm foods are recommended and sour foods are avoided, as these are said to act on the liver. Summer is also *yang*, and the heart is strong; Traditional Chinese Medicine principles recommend gentle foods, and to avoid bitter foods as these might impact on the heart. Autumn is considered good for the growth of *yin*; at this time people are advised to avoid hot and strong foods (acrid foods) and to increase sour foods, as acrid foods are said to act on the lungs while sour foods apparently help the liver during this season. Winter is the time for preserving *yin* and preparing *yang*, thus warm foods are encouraged and salty foods avoided, as acrid foods are said to act on kidneys, which are *yang* and should be preserved in winter.

Harmonising hot or cold constitutions

According to a 50-year-old woman in Sydney (originally from Hong Kong), two types of bodily constitution are classified:

> If you are a 'hot' type, you should eat some cool food. On the other hand, if you belong to the 'cold' type, you should eat some 'hot' food. I think *yin* and *yang* belongs to something like that.

Chinese people commonly refer to 'hot' and 'cold' types. Foods of the opposite nature are generally used to balance the type. A 'hot' or *yang* person should eat lighter, cool *yin* foods in order to preserve the body. Food in this category includes fruit, vegetables, beans and eggs, which are easily digested and transformed into *qi* and blood. In order to balance a *yin* or 'cold' type, a person should keep warm and 'hot' for which purpose *yang* foods are recommended. Generally, *yang* foods consist of animal meats such as beef or lamb and spicy plants such as ginger and pepper.

A 28-year-old man in Brisbane (originally from Vietnam) voiced similar concerns about these hot and cold types:

> When we talk about eating, my parents may talk about pyretic *qi* (熱氣). If we have it, my parents would prepare some cool foods. Sometimes, we may need some therapeutic food to balance our bodies.

Young men are thought to have a relative excess of *yang*, the symptoms of which Traditional Chinese Medicine would say include a hoarse voice and pimples. An excess of *yang* is also referred to as too much heat or 'pyretic *qi*'. In Traditional Chinese Medicine, this signifies fire and heat in the lungs and stomach, and a deficit of *yin*. Foods that are said to contribute to 'pyretic *qi*' belong to the deep-fried, roasted and spicy groups. The remedy for Traditional Chinese Medicine is to take soups that contain *yin* ingredients to cool the body and counteract *yang* excess. Cool foods are those that require less processing and handling such as steamed foods, fruit and vegetables.

Tonic therapy helps to maintain a balance of *yin* and *yang*, by strengthening vital energy with *yang*, and nourishing blood with *yin*. *Nei Jing* has the following explanation (*Plain Questions*, chapter 5:43):

> When the disease is caused by deficiency of vital energy and blood, the vital energy and blood can be restored using tonic therapy.

Traditional Chinese Medicine recognises four types of physical constitution (Flaws 1994:32–33):

- Wood or fire constitutions are characterised by strong-willed, aggressive or nervous dispositions. People in their twenties, thirties and forties are prone to this type of constitution.
- Phlegmatic or damp constitutions refer to the body accumulating phlegm or dampness as a result of a weak spleen and poor stomach function.

- *Yin*-deficient types are likely to be middle-aged people. By the age of forty years, in Traditional Chinese Medicine theory, *yin* would be reduced by half as a result of *yin* and *yang* activity.
- *Yang*-deficient types are likely to be older or elderly people. The *yang* energy wanes at this time of 'fire at the gate of life', manifesting in the body as a slowing of metabolism and a reduction in body heat.

People can also be born *yang*-deficient. *Nei Jing* (*Spiritual Pivot*, chapter 72:779) describes the different types of man with *yin* and *yang* constitutions. A man with much *yang* appears 'relax[ed], gay, and satisfied', a man with little *yang*, 'tosses his head when standing and sways when walking', a man with little *yin* is 'cool and shallow, he likes to injure others', and a man with much *yin* becomes, 'solemn, but he is modest in consciousness'.

It is important to know that the above categories are only general guidelines and are not fixed. Diagnosing *yin* and *yang* constitutions is a complicated matter and people fall into the trap of oversimplifying and stereotyping (Hammer 1990). Instead of using *yin* and *yang* to designate whether one is strong or weak, healthy or sick, it is considered more appropriate to use descriptions of *how* one is strong, weak or sick (Beinfield & Korngold 1991).

Disease resulting from imbalance

Three contributive factors are considered to cause disease: external *yang* factors including climatic, infectious and contagious influences; internal dysfunctions referred to as *yin* factors; and accidental and traumatic injuries, which are partly *yin* and *yang* (Ho & Lisowski 1993:18).

Some participants attributed the causes of disease to wind, dampness, heat, and cold, in accordance with Traditional Chinese Medicine belief regarding the six pathogenic external factors of dryness, dampness, cold, summer-heat, wind and rain, or the internal disharmony of *yin* and *yang*, stress, improper diet and an unbalanced life (*Nei Jing*, *Spiritual Pivot*, chapter 44). Traditional Chinese Medicine theory argues that under normal conditions, our bodies can adjust to those external seasonal changes, but not if they are in excess or deficiency; once these seasonal changes become the six evils, they can lead to disease. In the case of a weak constitution without strong bodily defences, the evils may attack the body through the skin, mouth and nose (Lin & Flaws 1991:99).

For example, when the Severe Acute Respiratory Syndrome (SARS) outbreak occurred in early 2003, this condition was considered in Traditional

Chinese Medicine as a 'hot' condition triggered by the wetness or humidity of spring. The 'heat toxin' and 'dampness' were said to be weakening the lung *qi* or vital energy; as a result, fluid accumulated in the lungs (*Wall Street Journal*, May 8 2003:B.1).

Due to wind

In Traditional Chinese Medicine, wind is commonly believed to create disharmony in the body. In the *Historical Records* (史記) compiled by Sze-ma Tsien (司馬遷 c. 90 BCE), the concept of 'wind' as the causative factor for illness was introduced in a report on the clinical presentations of the physician, Shun-yu Yi, as 'wind attacking the kidney' (Bowers & Purcel 1974:6). Wind is the most destructive of all 'diseases' according to *Nei Jing* (*Plain Questions*, chapter 9:106): 'Disease elicit[ed] by wind evil [occupies] the first place of all diseases'. In Traditional Chinese Medicine, wind is considered capable of penetrating the body's surface and assisting the entry of other adverse forces, namely dampness, dryness, cold, and heat (Beinfield & Korngold 1991).

A 45-year-old man in Armidale (originally from Beijing), had the following experience of wind attack while he lived in Beijing:

> In the view of Traditional Chinese Medicine, if you sit all the time facing into the wind, you run the risk of being paralysed. There were cases like this in northern China. Facial paralysis is not commonly seen in Australia.

This man postulated that wind could cause facial paralysis. According to *Nei Jing*, wind 'attack' can affect three parts of our bodies – the upper, middle and lower parts – and the energies of the three parts are different. When one's body is weak and experiences wind attack, the disease will start in the upper parts.

Facial paralysis is referred to as 'wind stroke' (中風) in Traditional Chinese Medicine. Wind [evil] can easily invade when the body is weakened, such as by a lack of *qi* or blood as well as by worry, anger, improper diet, excessive sex, or attack by external evils. The blockage of *qi* and blood may manifest as a sudden deviation of the face (Flaws 1994).

The wind category is divided into wind–heat and wind–cold, which differentiate different symptoms. According to the explanation in *Nei Jing* (*Plain Questions*, chapter 3:23), the nature and causes of cold and heat are produced through exposure to wind and dew. Wind is regarded as *yang* evil which produces heat; and dew is *yin* evil which produces cold; thus, the syndrome of cold and heat occurs.

A wind–heat attack was related by an 87-year-old woman in Sydney (originally from Taiwan):

> I had dizziness and headache due to the attack of wind, the so-called wind–heat syndrome (風熱症) by Traditional Chinese Medicine. I could not open my eyes and I had a migraine.

In Traditional Chinese Medicine, headache is a symptom of 'wind–heat attack' and manifests as a type of common cold with pronounced high fever, severe headache and swollen throat. Some attacks are said to start as a 'wind cold' which may progress to so-called wind–heat. Another explanation for headache in Traditional Chinese Medicine involves the liver. If it is overtaxed and 'heat' is generated, the blood becomes hot and heat rises and flows toward the head, causing a headache (Hammer 1990).

The wind–cold experience was associated with insufficient rest following childbirth by a 48-year-old woman in Sydney (originally from Hong Kong). During her resting month, she continued working and moving house. After that, her hands and legs suffered from malfunction and she was in pain all over her head, hands and legs:

> You got what Traditional Chinese Medicine calls 'wind–cold' when you get wet during your resting month, that is, not having sufficient nourishing food intake and working too hard.

In Traditional Chinese Medicine, diseases of the upper part of the body are said to be caused by wind–cold. If a woman is deprived of the rest and good food recommended for replenishing her body during her 'resting month' following a birth, it is believed the constitution will be weakened and become prone to attacks of wind and cold. As such, 'when evil *qi* attacks, there is emptiness of *qi*,' and 'when the constitution is empty, there is a lack of ability to defend, and wind, cold, and damp evil will cause *bi* [as pronounced in Chinese, meaning blockage]' (Flaws 1994:133). The blockage of *qi* and blood caused by wind, cold and wetness is thought to be manifested as pain in various parts of the body.

Due to heat

In Western biomedical thinking, heat is associated with increased metabolic activity and circulation; excessive heat equates with inflammation and fever (Beinfield & Korngold 1991). According to Traditional Chinese Medicine theory, however, excessive heat in the body is not necessarily synonymous with a high body temperature. Chinese people commonly refer to 'pyretic *qi*' (熱氣), meaning excessive heat in the body after having too much *yang* food such as fried and spicy foods. Pyretic *qi* manifests as dryness in the mouth, sore throat, skin allergies and constipation. This concept of pyretic *qi* was expressed by a 74-year-old woman in Sydney (originally from See Yup, Mainland China).

Traditional Chinese Medicine is good for eliminating pyretic *qi* and dampness in the body. The symptoms of damp heat are constipation or feeling heat in the rectum, stomach pain, and yellowish sputum.

According to Traditional Chinese Medicine principles, dampness usually combines with cold, heat, or wind. Damp–heat symptoms are manifested by painful swellings, inflammations, sores, abscesses or ulcers with pus. Foods such as sugar or fatty or fried foods are thought to cause damp heat. Constipation in Traditional Chinese Medicine is attributed to fire and heat, deficient *yin* and too much *yang*. The feelings of heat in the rectum and stomach pains are signs of a damp–heat attack.

A 32-year-old woman in Brisbane (originally from Papua New Guinea) thought Western people are perhaps not susceptible to pyretic *qi*:

> My parents talk about pyretic *qi* all the time. I do not know why I have more nose-bleeds than my Australian friends, they never have them. My parents say I eat too much fried foods or chocolate. They gave me a Traditional Chinese Medicine powder preparation.

This woman was brought up in the West. She compared the nature of her bleeding nose with the experience of her Western friends, who perhaps ate the same foods but did not get nose-bleeds. However her parents, seeing her nose-bleeds as a sign of pyretic *qi* brought on by too much fried foods and chocolate, gave her Traditional Chinese Medicine as a remedy.

A 71-year-old man in Brisbane (originally from Papua New Guinea) also cited fried foods as a cause of pyretic *qi*. Chinese people traditionally attribute any discomfort, such as a sore throat or adverse reactions, to excessive heat (pyretic *qi*). This man believed Western people were perhaps not susceptible to 'pyretic *qi*' after consuming fried foods because they drank lots of beer, which is a *yin* food, helping to balance the excessive yang of fried foods.

> Pyretic *qi* is very common among my generation and the next generation. We hand this Traditional Chinese Medicine concept down to the next

generation. Western people have the habit of eating fried foods, but they drink lots of beer which is a cool type of food.

The concept of accumulated heat inside one's body being the cause of skin disorders such as pimples and blackheads was cited by a 62-year-old practitioner of Traditional Chinese in Sydney (originally from Mainland China). In his opinion, the treatment purpose of Traditional Chinese Medicine is to clear the accumulated heat inside the lungs and spleen. A 21-year-old man in Brisbane (originally from Hong Kong) shared this view. He had been told by a practitioner in Traditional Chinese Medicine that his dermatitis (skin disorder) was due to too much heat, and had been advised to use Traditional Chinese Medicine to get rid of the toxins in his body.

The concept of 'heat' was further explored by a 45-year-old man in Armidale (originally from Beijing, Mainland China):

> I find Traditional Chinese Medicine concepts sound unreal, such as heat... For example, in Traditional Chinese Medicine watermelon is cold; you can eat it when you have heat. Traditional Chinese Medicine is good to get rid of the heat from our bodies. Western medicine does not talk about heat. Traditional Chinese Medicine divides heat into different types of heat: strong heat, weak heat, *yin* heat, *yang* heat.

This man acknowledged that some concepts in Traditional Chinese Medicine are difficult to grasp, and 'sound unreal'. Explanations for strong heat, and weak heat, *yin* heat and *yang* heat can be found in Beinfield and Korngold (1991). According to them, all healthy organs produce 'strong heat' that helps to combat stagnation. For example, at the early stage of distress and at later stages of stress, 'weak heat' develops. 'Weak heat' refers to heat in the body caused by long-term disease, which weakens the body and causes it to overheat. A person can experience *yin* heat and *yang* heat in their body at the same time. For example, weak heat or *yin* heat in the kidney is said to produce heat that is manifested as weak sweat. Heat in the hands and in the feet as *yang* heat is linked profuse perspiration. This strong manifestation of *yang* is attributed to high physical activity, fever or warm spicy foods.

Harmony in living

Chinese philosophy is centred on the harmonious human relationships recommended in *I Ching* and in Confucian and Taoist teachings. This section is concerned with the various contexts under which one employs strategies for harmonious living. This philosophy of living is socially and culturally located, and is related to significant others and society. In Chinese societies, discourses on the philosophy of living are prominent (Lam & Wong 1995). One of the chief characteristics is the emphasis on balance and harmony in life. The principles are well documented in *Chung Yung* (or *The Doctrine of the Mean*, 400–500 BCE) of Confucianism, and are emphasised in Taoism, providing a significant basis for Traditional Chinese Medicine.

The Chinese word *Chung* (中) means 'in the middle' (China was referred to in ancient times as the 'Middle Kingdom') or 'equilibrium'. *Yung* means 'common or ordinary' or 'harmony'. In chapter 1 of *Chung Yung* (*The Doctrine of the Mean*) the terms used in that treatise are defined. 'Equilibrium' is explained as 'no stirring' of emotions, and 'harmony' is to act in 'due degree' (in a proper manner). Section five states that when equilibrium and harmony is achieved, 'a happy order will prevail throughout heaven and earth, and all things will be nourished and flourish'. Moreover, harmony recognises differences and co-existence, as pointed out in chapter 30 (my translation):

> All things nurture together without harming each other.
> Each pursues its own way without opposing each other.
> … It is this which makes heaven and earth so great.

The philosophical roots of Traditional Chinese Medicine commonly refer to balance and harmony – between man and nature, between man and society, or between man and man. Such beliefs have been strongly influenced by Taoist philosophies regarding harmony. Chapter 4 of *Tao Te Ching* (trans. Cleary 1998:10) illustrates harmony in this way:

> The way is unimpeded harmony… It blunts the edges, resolves the complications, harmonises the light, assimilates to the world.

The clear message in *Tao Te Ching* is to make things easy and simple and to live peacefully in this world. The beauty of this quotation is reflected in the phrase 'harmonises the light, assimilates to the world' (和其光，同其塵), which means that one who is knowledgeable would not try to show off but would remain humble and hard-working in this world.

Other guides for harmony in living in *Tao Te Ching* include teaching us to take life easy (chapter 37), to be humble (chapters 6, 28, 34), to be contented (chapter 12), to follow nature (chapters 7, 25, 37), to do things properly and to eschew extremes (chapters 9, 12). The concept of balance has the aim of living a positive, receptive, honest, and happy life. Taoist philosophy teaches people to lead healthy and balanced lives through self-practice or development of self.

The concept of taking care of the self was reflected in Taoist practices such as social relationships, physical and mental health, balance, careful dieting and living, appropriate exercise, and preservation of energy (Yiu 1984). Needham (1974) described the art of the Taoist philosophy of living, including a list of techniques for mental and bodily hygiene in all aspects of living: proper dieting, moderation in everything, abandonment of all passions, preservation of energy, proper breathing techniques, mild exercise, and conservation of secretions. Taoists deeply believe that man's life depends on his own actions, and that he can make a better life for himself.

The importance of balance for health was illustrated through the 'care of the self' philosophy of life discussed by participants in the study. Aspects of this philosophy include understanding the role one is assigned to play in life, maintaining the natural flow, thinking deeply rather than superficially, and searching for truth.

Understanding my role assigned by Heaven

A 77-year-old man in Sydney (originally from Shanghai, Mainland China) conceived harmony as adhering to his role assigned by Heaven:

> I can say I have no trouble now and I am free from worries, one of the main components of Traditional Chinese Medicine. The main principle that guides harmony in life is to understand one's role assigned by Heaven. Thus I am no longer 'a frog watching the sky in a well'.

The identification with Heaven is typical of Taoism (chapter 25 of *Tao Te Ching*), in which all values and order on earth are seen to come from 'Heaven'. What this man considered important regarding Traditional Chinese Medicine was the balancing concept that helped him to be free from worry and to expand his horizons so that he no longer felt claustrophobic, 'a frog watching the sky in a well' (井底之蛙). Chuang Tzu (399–295 BCE), the great Taoist and Chinese philosopher, explained being 'free from worries' as a means of transcending emotional disturbance and achieving 'peace of spirit' (Fung 1973).

For this 77-year-old man, the main principle that guides a balanced life is understanding one's role, that is, when to advance and when to retreat in the proper way. When young he led 'an emperor's life' in which everything was given to him. He had all sorts of sumptuous, nutritious Traditional Chinese Medicine foods. He had no worries and did not have to stretch his intellect: 'I did not know how high the sky was and how deep the earth was' (不知天有多高地有多深).

In time, he faced great upheavals in his society (the Chinese revolution in 1949 and the Cultural Revolution in the 1960s), and his life changed from one of plenty to one of simplicity. He adjusted well amid the turmoil; he said 'simple tea and rice save[d] my life'. This quotation illustrates the principles of simple contentment, adaptability and not going to extremes, as proposed by the balancing and harmonious concepts developed in *The Doctrine of the Mean* and Taoist teachings. He learnt how to take care of his body by simple means and to disregard the trivialities of life. As he said, 'what is gone is gone; you have to focus on today', reflecting the Chinese philosophy that emphasises this present world, which is practical and realistic.

'Heaven' is mentioned again, along with the balancing concepts of keeping calm and peaceful, taking life easy, and not focusing on the unpleasant past, by a 76-year-old man in Sydney (originally from See Yup, Mainland China):

Traditional Chinese Medicine soup is very important for Chinese people. Elderly Chinese people in China have gone through 'wind and rain' (風風雨雨).We shouldn't think of anything bad but should talk about good things, 'Heaven falls down like being covered by a blanket (天跌下來像毯子蓋).

'Heaven falling like being covered by a blanket', a common saying among Chinese people, refers to how one can remain calm in mind and attitude during times of disaster. This man's philosophy of living embraced physical and spiritual dimensions. To care for himself physically, he used Traditional Chinese Medicine soups along with having regular check-ups with his Western doctor. He made use of the Australian environment to exercise regularly. Importantly, he maintained a balanced mind. 'Wind and rain' refers to the turmoil of life. People of his age, in his experience, would have experienced great turmoil in life such as wars and revolutions. In spite of the hardships of his life, he was able to live happily and contentedly. His strategy was to focus on pleasant things and the present moment. Above all, the attitudes of pacifism and tolerance enabled him to lift his everyday life into a more creative and healthy form of living.

Lifting the gate of sewage

People practice Qi Gong, an exercise regime associated with Traditional Chinese Medicine, in order to achieve harmony of living. A 62-year-old male practitioner of Traditional Chinese Medicine in Sydney (originally from Mainland China) had a firm belief in following nature and adhering to a health regime of practising Qi Gong:

> Qi Gong exercise helps us to relax and follow the way of nature, which is like 'the gate of the sewage being lifted up', allowing for drainage of the natural flow.

He referred metaphorically to the balance and natural flow of *qi*, which is the basis for maintaining health. He used two further metaphors to convey his philosophies of living centring on the body. He spoke of Qi Gong as helping to follow 'the way' of nature, a Taoist expression. Again, Chuang Tzu (399–295 BCE) explained the meanings of nature as understanding and harmonising with nature, and ensuring happiness and goodness.

This 62-year-old man also spoke of the body as a 'storehouse', implying that careful attention was needed to maintain balance and avoid excess in order to function well. Accumulated excesses should be purged, and only what is needed should be kept:

> The body is likened a storehouse. There were goods [foods] already in store ten years ago which you could not sell, yet you keep on adding new goods. You should empty the storehouse – sell what you can sell, eat what you can eat. If you cannot eat so much, give some to your friends.

He used further body metaphors to link body parts with action:

> Your gallbladder should be big and your heart should be small (膽大心小) in action.

The 'gallbladder' being big refers to having great courage, and a 'small heart' refers to undertaking work with meticulous care. Taken together, he was saying the process of change would require great courage and meticulous action.

Seeing more with closed eyes

In the view of a 40-year-old woman in Armidale (originally from Beijing, Mainland China), her concept of balance in health related to Chinese exercise and she recommended the following:

One can see more things when you close your eyes than when you open your eyes while practicing Chinese exercise, which aims at 'slow movement' and building 'inner calmness' to regulate us.

She implies that when your eyes are closed you can think deeply and maintain balance more easily; when you open your eyes you see only the superficial world. Traditional Chinese Medicine exercise emphasises 'refining and cultivating your character', 'calmness' and slowness, which brings balance to our hearts.

Chinese philosophy tends to be self and inwardly directed. In *The Doctrine of the Mean*, cultivating one's own character is seen as the first step toward governing others: 'Knowing how to cultivate his own character, he knows how to govern other men (Book 20, chapter 11). In the same classic, a 'superior man' is seen as being quiet and calm (Book 14, chapter 4).

Searching for truth in life

A 45-year-old man in Sydney (originally from Hong Kong) also used Qi Gong exercise in pursuing his philosophy of living:

> I started Chinese exercise to search for the meanings of life. What is the purpose of life? All I needed was to refine and cultivate my character. Chinese exercise helped me to practice my patience, so I could be a good man.

According to Max Weber, human beings are suspended in webs of meanings they have spun (Geertz 1975; Yu 1994). The search for the meaning of life is particularly important during spiritual suffering, in which the meaningful webs become insecure and shaken; thus human beings constantly try to spin the web.

Regarding patience, there is a Chinese saying that a 'hundred patience turns into gold'(百忍成金). This man viewed patience as a virtue and as a basis for harmonious social relationships. This 'patience' was emphasised in the traditional Chinese family system, which provided 'a training school' for mutual tolerance (Lin 1977:45). In the traditional Chinese family, obedience was the rule and patience a necessity. There was little room within the family for unfettered individual expression; people tended to follow others' ideas and take things for granted.

Surpassing Traditional Chinese Medicine: keeping busy

An 80-year-old woman in Sydney (originally from Taiwan) presented a different case. She did not use Traditional Chinese Medicine to nourish her body, but instead had worked out a regime of care for both her physical and spiritual needs. She insisted on keeping busy doing gardening, otherwise, she would 'feel crippled'. She was careful about what she ate, keeping to simple good quality foods, such as vegetables she had grown herself, and a little meat. On the moral level, she suggested:

> Do not think too much, be satisfied, and have a loving heart – loving, honest, and peaceful. The moral of living is not to cause trouble, to live in harmony, to take life easy, and not to be boastful.

Some of the characteristics of Chinese philosophy are reflected in the qualities she recommended. 'The loving heart' reflects Confucian teachings in benevolence or *yen*. 'Harmony' in *The Doctrine of the Mean* is the Tao's balancing concept of being 'not extreme but harmonious'. Being satisfied with life can be traced to Lao Tzu, whose maxim was 'one who is contented is always rich' (*Tao Te Ching*, chapter 33). This participant's philosophy of living would have lead her to be in perfect harmony with herself and others; and her happiness in life derived from simple means – the cultivation of her inner virtuous self.

Reflections

Balance in *yin* and *yang* suggests interaction between *yin* and *yang*, with all the characteristics of co-existence, change and transformation which adhere to the laws of nature. Balance in *yin* and *yang* therapy aims to restore equilibrium; an excess or deficiency of either is believed to predispose a person to illness. Imbalances in life are said to cause imbalances in the body, stress, and blockage of *qi*. Negative emotional factors also upset the *yin* and *yang* equilibrium, but this is not likely with positive emotional factors.

Foods are classified into *yin* and *yang* types according to the principles of Traditional Chinese Medicine. *Yin* foods are used for blood building in females and *yang* foods for building vital energy in males. *Yin* and *yang* foods should be consumed with regard to individual constitutions and used in conformity with the seasons.

Congruent with Traditional Chinese Medicine principles, some participants considered wind and heat to be the main causes of bodily imbalance. According to Traditional Chinese Medicine, the main effect of excessive wind and heat on the body is the blockage of the natural flow of *qi* or vital energy. Excessive wind was cited as the cause of facial paralysis;

wind–heat as the cause of headache; and wind–cold as the cause of physical discomfort due to lack of rest and insufficient intake of good foods during the resting month. Excessive heat is referred to as 'pyretic *qi*', which manifests as constipation as a result of having too much *yang* food (such as fried or spicy foods). Participants also pointed out that their Western friends did not appear to suffer from 'pyretic *qi*' even after eating fried foods. A reason given for this was the consumption of beer, a cool type of food, which helps to balance the heat effect of fried foods.

A key feature of Traditional Chinese Medicine is that it relates closely to harmony in living. Participants positively engage themselves in the care of self, aiming for balance and harmony. The philosophical underpinnings, including adhering to nature, taking life easy, being calm, quiet, patient and humane, and living in harmony are all important parts of participants' quests for healthy living.

And finally a case was presented where Traditional Chinese Medicine did not play a significant part in a participant's life, illustrating a life in balance. In this case harmony in life was maintained without the aid of Traditional Chinese Medicine through positive engagement with life and health-promoting activities.

The following chapter reveals the significance of Traditional Chinese Medicine in the three stages of life: youth, adulthood, and old age.

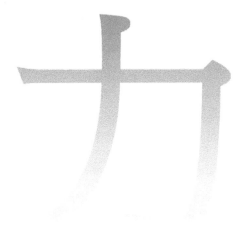

chapter five

Youth, Adulthood and Old Age

(Pronounced as *li*, which refers to strength in youth, adulthood, and old age)

A balance between the physical and moral integrity of people lays the
foundation for a strong and healthy nation.

Dr Sun Yat-sen (Sun 1963)

Introduction

Good health was considered the greatest blessing in ancient Chinese texts
(Yiu 1984) such as *Sheung Shu* (尚書), the oldest Chinese history, which
was recorded in the Zhou Dynasty (1027–221 BCE) (Lau 1978). Traditional
Chinese Medicine embraces the fundamental concept of *qi* as the vital energy
which permeates our lives. Historically, health was combined with bodily
integrity and moral living. For an individual, vigour in health commonly refers
to exuberant and resilient strength of body or mind. In Sun Yat-sen's view, a
balance between the physical and moral integrity of a nation's people lays the
foundations for a strong and healthy nation (Sun 1963). In the book *Nei Jing*
(or *Yellow Emperor's Canon of Internal Medicine*), the strength of a human body

is referred to as the essence of life – the foundation of man. Many references in *Nei Jing*, the first Chinese medical classic (Tang Dynasty 618–907 CE) reflect the Tao's *yin* and *yang* concepts of balance, following nature, and preserving vitality in traditional Chinese health care. For example, good health was achieved through *yin* and *yang* balance producing a strong body and spirit:

> If the *yin* and *yang* energies of a man are kept in a state of equilibrium, his body will be strong, his spirit sound. If his *yin* and *yang* energies fail to balance, his vital energy will decline until finally exhausted.
>
> (*Plain Questions*, chapter 3:22)

Good health was maintained through a regular pattern of life following nature, with no indulgence in sexual pleasures because this would deplete the vigour in a body:

> Those who knew the way to keep good health… in accordance with nature… They were able to modulate their daily life in harmony with the way of recuperating the essence and vital energy… indulge in sexual pleasures and use up their vital energy and ruin their health.
>
> (*Plain Questions*, chapter 1:7)

This view also appears in the classical Western tradition, as exemplified by Aristotle who suggested moderation and the avoidance of extremes in order 'to locate the mean and cultivate practical wisdom and temperance' (Gabardi 2001:145).

For the Chinese, energy can be divided into *yin* energy and *yang* energy, which serve different needs. According to *Nei Jing* (trans. Wu and Wu 1999):

> For human beings, those who draw support from *yang* energy abundantly are men and consist of vital energy; those who draw support from *yin* energy abundantly are women and are for blood.
>
> (*Plain Questions*, chapter 5:38)

Traditional Chinese Medicine is perceived as strength and energy by Chinese people of all ages, young, middle-aged and elderly, uncovering deep-rooted cultural meanings. *Yang* energy is the basis for boys' vitality and adult male virility, and *yin* energy is for female nourishment and building blood.

Vitality during youth sets the stage for preventive health – building strength in boys for their manhood and preparing girls for healthy motherhood.

For male adults, Traditional Chinese Medicine is associated with sexually orientated energy; the seminal essence, the main source of male vitality, is directed toward virility and power for men. For women, Traditional Chinese Medicine is directed toward maximising fertility and childbearing capacity.

In old age, preserving health and maintaining *qi* (energy) are more important. Through self-efficacy, striving to live with the utmost strength and seeking to live a long and productive life, people maintain continuity with the past while also creating a better future.

Traditional Chinese Medicine for boys

Historically, the Chinese people held their children in high esteem. Confucian teaching strongly advocated caring for children. Children were considered important because of their importance for future generations:

> The Master said: A youth is to be regarded with respect. How do we know that his future will not be equal to our present?
>
> (*Analects*, Book 9, chapter 22)

In terms of physical strength, which in youth was not yet considered to be fully formed, Confucius advised the young not to indulge in sexual gratification: 'In youth, when the physical powers are not yet settled, he guards against lust' (*Analects*, Book 16, chapter 7). This was congruent with the idea that improper sexual desires would strip men of their most precious possessions – seminal essence, or semen, thus depleting them of energy in health and reproductive potential.

For parents, the health of their children is a primary concern, as a strong constitution is considered the basis for a child being productive and useful in the future. In this study, the role of Traditional Chinese Medicine for the energy of boys is focused in the areas of enhancing learning, strengthening *yang* for a productive future, and preventing disease or ill-health.

Enhancing learning

A 45-year-old man in Armidale (originally from Beijing) recalled his youthful experience of Traditional Chinese Medicine for enhancing learning:

> When I was a child, Traditional Chinese Medicine was used for natural therapy. Food similar in appearance would nourish the similar parts of the body (以形補形). If we eat brains, it was believed we would be clever... We also ate liver, good for building blood, and heart for nourishing our heart.

The doctrine of similarity is discerned here – body parts are considered to be nourished by food or medicinal items of similar appearance and analogous function to those body parts (Anderson 1988). Eating brains is believed to improve intelligence, liver to build blood, and heart to improve cardiac function. In Traditional Chinese Medicine, the brain is linked to the heart, liver and kidneys. The liver also corresponds to emotions, and the heart is considered to control conscious and mental activities (Lin & Flaws 1991). Health-building foods are considered good for enhancing learning in young people, and learning is highly regarded in many Chinese societies. Confucius said, 'When I was fifteen, I set my mind on learning' (*Analects*, Book 2, chapter 4).

Strengthening yang in boys

For a 76-year-old man in Sydney (originally from See Yup, Mainland China), Traditional Chinese Medicine was closely related to strengthening *yang* energy for boys. He favourably recalled the following experience:

> I had Traditional Chinese Medicine, *cordyceps* (東蟲草), as a boy, which was not as expensive as now. My grandmother used to prepare this together with pork. That is good for boys' kidney energy (補腰腎).

The Traditional Chinese Medicine, *cordyceps*, is notable for its male (*yang*) strengthening properties. Kidneys, as this man pointed out, are significant in Traditional Chinese Medicine because of their links to male reproduction. People believe that the 'jing' essence, or semen, is stored in the kidneys. Kidney jing determines the growth of young people and is used for future reproductive function. However, kidney energy develops gradually and is not at its full potential in young people:

> For a male, his kidney energy becomes prosperous by the age of eight. By then, his hair develops and his permanent teeth emerge.

> His kidney energy becomes prosperous by the age of sixteen; he is filled with vital energy and is able to let out sperm...

> By the age of twenty-four, his kidney energy is well developed to reach the state of an adult.

> (*Plain Questions*, chapter 1:9)

'Kidney energy' develops according to an eight year cycle, and it is also responsible for the growth of bones. Kidney energy or jing is said to reach the well-developed stage of an adult at the age of twenty-four.

Yang foods are commonly prepared for boys in the form of soups, which makes Traditional Chinese Medicine more palatable especially for children. An example was given by a 50-year-old man in Armidale (originally from Taiwan) regarding his brothers and himself:

> Boys in my family were given Traditional Chinese Medicine around the age of ten to enhance strength. My parents used to prepare me soups to strengthen my health; soups like boiling chicken with Traditional Chinese Medicine.

Foods are divided into *yin* and *yang* foods. *Yang* foods such as meat are widely used to strengthen *yang*. This is congruent with the group interview data in Brisbane (with people who were originally from Taiwan). This group said a common practice in Taiwan is to give boys Traditional Chinese Medicine such as the Perfect Tenth tonic soup (十全大補湯), which helps them to grow stronger and taller. Again, they reported that Traditional Chinese Medicine for boys is often prepared with meat such as chicken or pork.

Other *yang* meats one can find in Australia are deer and sheep. Their tendons are reputed to be good for male strength, as noted by a 58-year-old woman in Sydney (originally from See Yup, Mainland China):

> For boys, people say that some Traditional Chinese Medicine helps to strengthen *yang*. In Australia, you can find many deer and sheep. Their tendons can be dried and used for the strength of males.

Underlying the use of Traditional Chinese Medicine for boys is the assumption that boys are more active and require more energy foods to sustain their energy requirements. A 70-year-old woman living in Sydney (originally from Mainland China) said that Traditional Chinese Medicine serves to supplement energy:

> My parents said boys needed more food to match with their greater energy output. They gave more Traditional Chinese Medicine foods to their sons because they were more active than girls.

Preventing disease in boys

For preventive health care, Traditional Chinese Medicine was again presented in the form of soup and shared at family or social gatherings, as recalled by a 45-year-old man in Sydney (originally from Hong Kong):

> I had herbal tea when I was a boy, and during summer we had east melon soup (東瓜) prepared with Traditional Chinese Medicine that you can get from the Chinese medicine shops. My mother said that it helped to relieve heat in your body in summer.

Traditional Chinese Medicine is commonly given in the form of herbal tea because of its convenience. East melon, a *yin* food with cooling properties, is a popular spring and summer Traditional Chinese Medicine soup in Hong Kong. East melon is taken in summer for dinner or as a dessert for 'relieving heat'. In the hot and humid Hong Kong summer, this soup is believed to relieve heat and dampness in the body.

'Heat' has a different meaning in this context. Many Chinese people believe that too much 'heating' of food – in the form of fried, hot and spicy foods – should be avoided, as foods such as these may cause sickness and discomfort such as sore throats and skin irritations.

Parents are generally concerned that boys will grow up tall and strong, to present a strong masculine image. Traditional Chinese Medicine foods are commonly used to safeguard boys' health, as observed by a 70-year-old woman in Sydney (originally from Singapore):

> Every age group needs different Traditional Chinese Medicine foods if you want your sons to grow up tall and strong. In addition, you have to give them plenty of love. After the age of twelve, I gave my son *tifuch* flowers (田七) to safeguard him against bruises.

The Traditional Chinese Medicine, *tifuch,* is believed to stop bleeding and relieve pain. It has a reputation for preventing bruises and clearing blood. Another point worthy of noting here is this woman's thoughts on the psychology of parenting boys, and her use of Traditional Chinese Medicine as a safeguard and preventative measure for health.

Traditional Chinese Medicine for men

Discourses in Traditional Chinese Medicine associate masculinity with male sexual performance, as expressed by enhancing kidney *yang* energy, and consuming food items of 'sexual organs' for energy. These discourses are grounded in cultural history in relation to sexual health, a key preoccupation of Traditional Chinese Medicine. In ancient times, Chinese people recognised the importance of sexuality for maximising life and continuing the family line, and were concerned to enrich their sexual energy (Straten & Koeppen 1983). According to texts in the *Analects* and the works of Mencius, sex was considered a natural part of life. In *Analects* (Book 4, chapter 17) it is stated: 'I have not seen one who loves virtue as he loves sex', and Mencius was quoted as saying, 'Eating food and having sex is the nature of human beings' (Ruan 1991).

Traditionally, Chinese attitudes towards sexual health were presented in a pragmatic, matter-of-fact manner (Zhang & Rose 1999:176). However, there were still plenty of taboos marginalising certain forms of sexuality, suggesting that the focus was on enhancing reproduction. The general guidelines for achieving sexual vigour discouraged wasting semen and encouraged sexual abstinence, which was said to preserve jing or semen, improve heath and longevity, and benefit the production of good offspring. Other guidelines included proper food, proper breathing and exercise. Optimal sexual health was based on the concept of harmonising with nature as advocated by the Tao (Needham 1983; Zhang & Rose 1999). The associations between power, strength, masculinity and virility are noteworthy in the discourses of participants using Traditional Chinese Medicine as a means for realising manhood in a masculine culture.

Strengthening yang in men

A 62-year-old man in Sydney (originally from See Yup, Mainland China) was concerned about exhausting the 'essences', which may impact on virility:

> Yes, there is Traditional Chinese Medicine for virility. If males have weak kidneys this will lead to impotence; even if they experience an erection that is not good enough. The purpose of Traditional Chinese Medicine is to strengthen the kidneys (or *yang*).

'Kidney energy' is believed to govern the sexual health of males, and kidneys may become weak and exhausted and experience the loss of kidney jing or semen due to too much sex (Lin & Flaws 1991:46). According to *Nei Jing* (*Plain Questions*, chapter 1:10), male bodies develop to their best condition at the age of thirty-two, at which time the full vigour of 'kidney energy' is realised. 'Kidney energy' declines at the age of forty, there is a 'deficiency' of kidney energy at the age of fifty-six, and kidney energy becomes 'weak' when men turn sixty-four. Therefore, well-regulated and harmonious conduct was recommended for sustaining the sexual vigour of males. As the above passage demonstrates, the purpose of Traditional Chinese Medicine is to nurture and foster sexual vigour by sustaining this 'kidney energy'.

Assimilating energy from sexual organs

In Traditional Chinese Medicine, food and medicines prepared from sexual organs were used to enhance virility in men, as articulated by a 35-year-old woman in Sydney (originally from Hong Kong):

> Males are more active. I heard there was Traditional Chinese Medicine for enhancing the sexual prowess of males, such as three tigers' penis wine [which is prepared by adding Traditional Chinese Medicine].

A similar belief was held by a 76-year-old man in Sydney (originally from See Yup, Mainland China):

> I do not have money to buy deer penis, which is very nourishing for males. My friend planted some *cordyceps,* and I tried to plant them in my garden.

Deer penis as used in Traditional Chinese Medicine is very expensive. *Cordyceps*, with its reputation of boosting male virility, is considered a substitute when one cannot afford an expensive Traditional Chinese Medicine.

A belief governing the use of foods for virility and sexual health is that people can draw on the energy of powerful creatures by consuming them, particularly the sexual organs (Anderson 1988). Powerful creatures, such as tigers, are seen as symbols of male power or virility. Consuming tiger carries the implication that the consumer is a real man who has conquered a dangerous and powerful animal. This is illustrated in the classic Chinese novel, *The Water Margin* (水滸傳), attributed to Shih Nai-an (施耐庵) and Lo Kuan-chung (羅貫中) in the twelfth century. One of the heroic characters described in this novel, Wu Song (武從), was depicted as a man of great courage and power who killed a tiger bare-handed.

Traditional Chinese Medicine supplements that use the sexual organs of animals such as the penises of sheep, deer and tiger for enhancing virility are widely promoted. China has a long history of using animal sexual organs for medicine and health. Needham (1983) suggested that the practice of the

Chinese using animal testes was first published in year 1253, in the book *Classical Fundamental Prescriptions of Universal Benefit.*

The Brisbane group (from Taiwan) shared this view about using the sexual organs of animals for male virility. This group suggested that Taiwanese people ate everything, including bears' paws, usually prepared with Traditional Chinese Medicine, in the belief that these items would strengthen male virility. Sexual organs, including penis of tiger, were also popular. This group reported that a recent popular discourse in Taiwan had been concerned with whether men's sexual organs were longer after consuming all those sexual organs. The group suggested, 'Chinese people believe what you eat will nourish the same part of your body', the doctrine of similarity.

(It is recognised that the demand for Traditional Chinese Medicine products such as bear bile, bear paw and tiger penis poses significant threats to some endangered species. A British health officials' report (Knight Ridder Tribune Business News 2006:1) found powdered rhino horns and tiger bones in some Traditional Chinese Medicine. In a study of 1000 of the most commonly used Traditional Chinese Medicine products, 10 contained ingredients from endangered species, and 80 per cent of the 13 000 ingredients were found to be derived from fauna and flora (Zhao Runhuai of China Material Company, reported in Liu 2000: 8). Encouraged by some international governments and interest groups, Chinese academic institutions are now researching alternative ingredients and the Chinese government is moving toward limiting the trade in endangered species for Traditional Chinese Medicine, such as by reducing the number of bear farms (M2 Presswire 2006:1).)

In the following, a 50-year-old woman in Sydney (originally from Hong Kong) learnt from her mother about using animal sexual organs for male fertility:

> My mother mentioned that if you want to have babies, your husband has to eat the penis of sheep or penis of deer, which are for men. In the traditional Chinese view, people thought infertility was a problem with men only, not women. Because my mother is a traditional woman, she only talked about penis of deer for men.

In this statement we encounter the theme of infertility being a men's problem. In the male-dominated Chinese society, information on sexual culture tends to be focused and biased toward men's health regimens and diets, presumably contributing to this belief that male potency dominates fertility (Zhang & Rose 1999:171).

In offering her advice for male virility, a 58-year-old woman in Sydney (originally from See Yup, Mainland China) suggested a well-balanced diet, nourishing Traditional Chinese Medicine to boost energy, and the encouragement of good character. She commented that if people lived an unbalanced lifestyle, such as by smoking and drinking, then even if they have no virility problems their offspring may have health issues such as bad temper. The assumption here was that not taking care of oneself could impact severely on future generations.

Traditional Chinese Medicine for girls

In Traditional Chinese Medicine, *yin* energy is related to blood, according to *Nei Jing* (*Plain Questions*, chapter 5:38). Blood is referred to as the ruling aspect of female energy (Furth 1987). Using Traditional Chinese Medicine for 'blood-building' is a common practice among Chinese populations in China, Hong Kong, Taiwan, Korea, Australia, New Zealand and the United States (Ludman, Newman & Lynn 1989). In this study, the theme emerged that Traditional Chinese Medicine is given for girls' vitality to prepare them for motherhood. Three areas of focus could be discerned: Traditional Chinese Medicine for preventing disease and ill-health, for nourishing *yin*, and for ensuring girls' reproductive capacity.

Preventing disease in girls

Chinese people hold the general notion that females should take care of their health while they are young in order to experience healthy aging. A 58-year-old woman in Sydney (originally from See Yup, Mainland China) commented:

> [If] females do not take care when they are young to have proper Traditional Chinese Medicine nourishment, when they get old they bear the consequences. For example, if you have the body of the Chinese east melon, and tofu, [it is not surprising that] you have a headache one day, and leg weakness the next...

'East melon'(東瓜) and 'tofu'(豆腐) are used as metaphors of bodily weakness. Chinese east melon is huge and strong on the outside, but empty inside. Tofu is also soft outside, and after long hours being cooked for tofu soup, it is also empty inside. Traditional Chinese Medicine is used as a means of safeguarding against developing these characteristics.

Some female Chinese people used Traditional Chinese Medicine with the aim of enhancing their reproductive health, particularly for blood-building. They used different practices (popular in their social environments when they were young) to prepare themselves for motherhood.

Traditional Chinese Medicine is divided into superior, medium, and lower class therapies. Superior traditional Chinese medicines function to supplement *qi* and boost vitality; they are used for preventive health care and are generally non-toxic. Ginseng and deer's antler belong to this category. Medium-class Traditional Chinese Medicine such as *pinellia* (半夏) is used for nourishing the body in chronic illness. Poke root, an example of a lower-class Traditional Chinese Medicine, is used for remedial treatment of acute or serious illness (Flaws 1994:88). For people who cannot afford the expensive Traditional Chinese Medicines, some substitutes can be used as health supplements.

A 74-year-old woman in Sydney (originally from See Yup, Mainland China) had the following experience with Traditional Chinese Medicine for nourishing her body:

> I ate the 13 days hen's eggs. They are eggs that have been incubated by hens for only 13 days. Inside the 13 days eggs you find the whole hen. People prepared it by adding some Traditional Chinese Medicine. My body was weak. How could we have the chance to try deer's antler and ginseng?

The woman was poor when she was young, and unable to afford the luxury of expensive Traditional Chinese Medicine, so instead she used the '13 days eggs' prepared with Traditional Chinese Medicine for blood-building. Some people believe that eating an egg with the whole chicken inside is very nutritious for the body. This is a common practice in the villages of southern China.

In contrast, a 35-year-old woman in Sydney (originally from Hong Kong) grew up in a comparatively prosperous home environment when she was young. Her father bought her various types of expensive Traditional Chinese Medicine when she was a teenager, apparently because she had poor blood circulation which manifested as 'cold' at puberty. In Hong Kong, Traditional Chinese Medicine is easily accessible and popular for therapeutic purposes. This woman was regularly given Traditional Chinese Medicine for preventive health care:

> I did not have any health problems except that my body was a bit 'cold'. At puberty, when I had my period I did not take much care of my body…

Later on, my father gave me ginseng, deer antler and white phoenix pills. I remember I started taking these when I was twelve or thirteen until the age of twenty.

A cold body was considered a sign of blood deficiency, and therefore warm foods were needed to build fitness and for future reproductive purposes. This principle is demonstrated in the following use of 'power soup' by a 30-year-old woman in Brisbane (originally from Papua New Guinea). She also considered Traditional Chinese Medicine as a preventive measure and for 'blood building'.

> I just knew the foods that I ate were different from Westerner's food… and so if you had too much fried foods you had to drink the soup… I think we had what we called 'power soup', I do not know what it was called, with lots of red little things in it.

In Papua New Guinea, where this woman was raised, a soup made with the Traditional Chinese Medicine of redmedler berries was used to nourish the blood, promote good health and benefit future reproductive function.

Nourishing yin *and reproduction*

Girls were given Traditional Chinese Medicine for nourishing *yin*, which was not fully developed in youth. Breasts were expected to serve the basic function of feeding growing babies, and Traditional Chinese Medicine was used to enhance them as in the following observation by a 50-year-old man in Armidale (originally from Taiwan):

> Girls in my family were given Traditional Chinese Medicine around the age of sixteen before marriage. Female is *yin*. Traditional Chinese Medicine was used for nourishing and beautifying the breasts for feeding babies.

In Chinese medical conception, the *yin* constitution is weakened during menstruation because of the loss of blood and during pregnancy (Furth 1987). In the following case, a 74-year-old woman in Sydney (originally from See Yup, Mainland China) used a nourishing Traditional Chinese Medicine to enrich her *yin* and to benefit reproduction.

> I took pills to nourish my *yin*. Because my period was not good, I had these pills before I had children. That was good for females.

The Traditional Chinese Medicine pills she mentioned were tiny pills contained in a thick 'plastic' round shells (smaller than a golf ball). The pills contained Traditional Chinese Medicine and black chicken, which was believed to be good for blood building. These Traditional Chinese Medicine pills were for long term therapeutic purposes.

Generational and geographic differences

Comparing data provides insight into the use of Traditional Chinese Medicine for girls across two different generations and from differing geographical backgrounds.

The middle-aged group in Brisbane (originally from Taiwan) suggested that Traditional Chinese Medicine for girls' vitality mainly targets reproduction and disease prevention. A common practice in Taiwan is to give girls Traditional Chinese Medicine so they can 'grow better and stronger'. Traditional Chinese Medicine such as *Four Ingredients Soup* (四物湯), and *Eight Ingredients Soup* (八珍湯) are given to girls around the age of ten to regulate their periods and to prepare them for child bearing.

The younger-aged group in Brisbane (originally from Hong Kong), however, held a different view. They considered that Traditional Chinese Medicine was more important for reinforcing 'good look' than for reproduction. Traditional Chinese Medicine had become a commodity in the commercialised female market in Hong Kong. These women viewed Traditional Chinese Medicine as being for 'body building', especially for 'enhancing breasts'. They preferred Traditional Chinese Medicine soups that were tasty, which they continued to take because of their availability in Brisbane. They did not find the *Four Ingredients Soup* and *Eight Ingredients Soup* mentioned by the middle-aged group in Brisbane particularly appealing because of the taste and dark colour of these soups.

Traditional Chinese Medicine for women

Discourses in Traditional Chinese Medicine concerning female vitality and reproduction were revealed through advice on fertility, the social meanings of fertility, and the practice of the resting month with its particular dietary practices for safeguarding future health.

Advice on fertility

A 62-year-old male practitioner of Traditional Chinese Medicine in Sydney (originally from Mainland China) gave the metaphor of a cold pool for an unproductive uterus:

Some women may have a 'cold uterus', which is likened to a cold pool; if you put baby fish in a cold pool they will all die. If you have a cold uterus you will not be able to conceive. The purpose of Traditional Chinese Medicine is to nourish *yin*.

A cold body is interpreted as having decreased 'body fire'. In women this manifests as a 'cold uterus', which is thought to affect fertility (Lin & Flaws 1991:45). To balance coldness, 'hot' *yang* foods are used. The importance of keeping warm and avoiding cold foods was expressed by a 58-year-old woman in Sydney (originally from Mainland China):

Traditional Chinese Medicine cannot control the sex of a baby but it can enhance the chances of fertility. Females have to keep warm, eat good foods, not eat cold foods, have good soups, and keep healthy and balanced. When the uterus is not cold, the chances of fertility are high.

Different areas of a balanced life are embraced for enhancing female fertility by using the metaphor of 'uterus' as incubator: keeping warm, which is a basic requirement for fertility; having warm and good foods; and living a balanced and healthy life. She continued by using a cake metaphor for making a baby, saying that to make good cakes one needs the right ingredients in sufficient quantities. For example, if not enough egg yokes and almonds are added, it would be impossible to make a good cake that was big and solid, and from this she drew a parallel to producing good children. She believed 'we are what we eat', that we need good foods to build up our bodies and thus enhance fertility.

Social meanings of fertility

Since a key goal of fertility is to continue the family line, preferably by producing a male heir, some Traditional Chinese Medicines are used in the belief that they will deliver a male child. Women experience social pressure to produce sons in male-dominated societies, as mentioned by a 40-year-old woman in Armidale (originally from Hong Kong). In her experience, she learnt of certain Traditional Chinese Medicine for having babies, especially some formulas for having boys that were well sought after. Having a boy first provides a woman with security and freedom from 'chasing' – pressure to become pregnant again until a boy has been produced.

However, there are signs that the preference for boys might be moderating. Based on his experience of living in a different city, a 39-year-old man in

Armidale (originally from Shanghai, Mainland China) stated that the sex of a child was not important in the big city where he used to live. The one-child policy of Mainland China may have had some influence on this traditional attitude, as compared with Hong Kong where boys are still preferred.

The 'resting month'

As mentioned earlier, pregnancy is considered a period of weakened constitutions. Generally, Chinese people believe it is important to have a 'resting month' (坐月) after delivering a baby, that is, a month of rest and recuperation in order to restore the energy of the body. This practice persists among Chinese people in Mainland China and Taiwan (Pillsbury 1978). Another purpose of this resting practice is to build up the body for future health. Without a good resting month after delivery, the stage would be set for poor health.

During this month, apart from having rest from other household work so as to focus on the newborn baby, a common practice is to prepare nourishing Traditional Chinese Medicine with meats such as chicken.

Sometimes, the quality of 'rest' a new mother gets signifies the amount of support she receives from other family members or perhaps from help employed to relieve the burden of running the household.

A 45-year-old man in Armidale (originally from Beijing) was fascinated by the large amounts of chicken consumed by women after delivery and especially during the resting month, remarking that 'women ate ten chickens, eighteen chickens, or twenty chickens'. He agreed that preparing chicken by boiling it in Traditional Chinese Medicine was good for building up a woman's blood and energy, which would be depleted after delivery. The body would be nourished both by the chicken and the supplements.

A 50-year-old woman in Sydney (originally from Hong Kong) spoke of her personal experience of a resting month. From her we have a description of 'vinegar ginger', constituted by pork leg, ginger and eggs together with sweet vinegar, a supplement believed to be good for women after childbirth. This becomes a social dish shared during visits to the mother and baby. She also had to avoid cold water and tried to have plenty of rest. Many elderly Chinese people hold the belief that one can contract rheumatic arthritis later in life if one touches too much cold water around the time of childbirth. The explanation for this is that an attack of pathogenic cold causes blockage of *qi* and blood, generating stagnation of a cold nature. This cold stagnation is manifested as pain, such as in the joints of the body (Xu 2001:61). In Traditional Chinese Medicine, *qi* and blood are considered mutually dependent and critical for the proper functioning and vitality of the body. The co-existence and interdependence of *qi* and blood are evident in the belief that blood can be transformed into *qi*, and that *qi* acts as a provider of blood.

The Brisbane group (originally from Taiwan) also recognised the importance of the resting month. The group pointed out two types of people that would benefit form Traditional Chinese Medicine. The first type was poor Chinese people in ancient days who had marginal nutrition and needed more nutritious foods. The second type was women after giving birth who would also need tonic foods to safeguard their future health. However, in this group's view, nutritional problems nowadays are different and eating too much meat is not good, so we should take simpler foods instead. Their explanation was that people no longer needed food supplements because foods are plentiful. Indeed, the upcoming generations were thought to suffer from excessive nutrition. However, for the older generation, the idea of taking food tonics to build up one's body when young persisted.

In one case, however, the idea of the resting month was rejected. A 32-year-old woman in Brisbane (originally from Papua New Guinea) did not hold such traditional ideas. She was more influenced by Western culture, and acted according to her own beliefs. She insisted on maintaining her personal hygiene and going out as usual during her resting month. Moreover, she continued to wash her hair during the resting month, rejecting the view this would put her at risk of 'wind' attacks that would weaken her body. Her understanding of why people had poor health in the past was that it was due to their lack of attention to hygiene.

Traditional Chinese Medicine for old age

Elderly Chinese people have long enjoyed high status and respect in Chinese societies. There is an old saying that 'an elderly person at home is like a treasure'(家有一老如有一寶). Confucian teachings advocated respect for elderly people: 'At home respect your parents. Away from home respect your elders' (Kelen 1983:22). The works of *Mencius* (*Liang Hiu Wang*, chapter 3:12) express due respect for the elderly at home and elsewhere: 'treat with the reverence due to age the elders in your own family, so that the elders in the families of others shall be similarly treated'. The idea that elderly people should be provided with a stable social environment so that they can enjoy healthy ageing is advised in the *Analects* (Book 5, chapter 5:6): 'In regard to the aged, give them repose'. In traditional Chinese thinking, it is considered a privilege to serve our aged parents. There is a deep sorrow when one's duty towards aged parents is not fulfilled while there was still opportunity. This attitude is reflected in the saying, 'The tree desires repose, but the wind will not stop; the son desires to serve but his parents are gone' (Lin 1938:1938).

Considering the privilege of being elderly, Chinese people in the past were content to look forward to old age, to enjoying being surrounded by children and grandchildren (兒孫滿堂). A common wish of the aged during a birthday party was to 'live to a hundred years old' (長命百歲). Therefore, maintaining the health of elderly people was seen to be of considerable importance, and extensive attention was paid to preserving health, maximising life and achieving immortality.

In the *Nei Jing,* the first five chapters are concerned with preserving health. Chapter 1 is a series of questions raised by the Yellow Emperor about the secret of healthy living, and the answers are given by the Taoist master Qibo. This example describes how ancient people lived so long by adhering to nature and maintaining their vigour:

> Their behaviour in daily life was all kept in regular patterns... They never overworked. In this way, they could maintain both the body and the spirit, and were able to live to the old age of more than one hundred years.
>
> (*Plain Questions*, chapter 1:7)

The message is clear concerning the importance attached to cultivating the body and the mind in order to preserve health and reach old age. Prolonged good health was believed to depend on discipline and moderation in eating, drinking and activities. Further advocacy for preserving health can be found in the Chinese medical treatise *The Thousand Golden Remedies* by Sun Si-miao (581–682 CE) (Ho & Lisowski 1993). Sun looked for ways to maintain health for he believed that human life is more precious than gold; once lost, it is lost forever (Yiu 1984:173). Sun's health advice included abstinence from sex to preserve semen, exercise, adaptation to the weather, and diet. Another prominent writer on health preservation was Lao Tzu, whose advice in the *Tao Te Ching* informed the analysis of the participants' views and the 'health regimes' that are described below.

Participants' discourses in Traditional Chinese Medicine for maintaining *qi* or strength in old age are revealing. They are linked to consistent adherence to health regimes and the positive relationship between Traditional Chinese Medicine and longevity.

Adhering to health regimes

An 80-year-old woman in Sydney (originally from See Yup, Mainland China) used Traditional Chinese Medicine as a means for achieving independence:

> Life is not predestined. Now I try to eat healthy foods, such as taking Traditional Chinese Medicine soup and exercise. It would be a great misery if one cannot take care of oneself. I do not mind living longer if I can be independent.

This attitude that 'life is not destined' reflects Taoist ideas that one's experience of life is not predetermined but is in one's own hands (Lam & Wong 1995:54), and that there is always something one can do to improve health such as by maintaining a healthy diet and exercise. A caring mother who lived with her son, this woman reported that she adhered to health regimes such as eating healthy Traditional Chinese Medicine soups and exercising, because she wanted to maintain her independence and did not want to become dependant on her son. She tried her best to be independent in spite of her advanced age. She used positive thinking and believed that through her actions she could improve her health.

An 87-year-old woman in Sydney (originally from Taiwan) reflected on what health meant to her:

> My view of health is 'free from pressure, and to be contented'. If you are contented, you will be happy. You should not think of anything negative and bad. I do not think too much, and I am satisfied.

This 70-year-old woman also in Sydney (originally from Singapore) revealed a similar line of thought:

> I gave up Qi Gong because I had a hip replacement. I think one ought to be contented all the time and enjoy life. There are always people better off than me, and there are people worse off than me. I always try to maintain a healthy life.

In the thinking of these elderly people are the common themes of 'do not think too much' and 'be contented', both of which reflect Taoist principles for preserving health. Lao Tzu suggests simplicity, minimising private thoughts, erasing greediness, and being contented and happy, as reflected in *Tao Te Ching* (trans. Lau 1963):

> Exhibit the unadorned and embrace the uncarved block,
> Have little thought of self and as few desires as possible.

> (*Tao Te Ching,* chapter 19)

'Do not think too much', that is, achieving a tranquil mind, is also encouraged in *Nei Jing*:

> Those who have a quiet spirit, their primordial energy will be moderate; their desires can be satisfied easily if only they are not insatiably greedy... As they have a quiet and stable state of mind, no desire can seduce their eyes, and no obscenity can entice their heart... thus, they are all able to live according to the way of keeping good health.

> (*Plain Questions*, chapter 1:8)

The above quote links certain mental states and desires with physical health, advising readers to restrain their greed in order to maintain a 'quiet mind' and preserve their 'vital energies'. When free from worldly gain and loss, one can be contented and happy. The way to gain harmony in life is believed to be by minimising worry and being contented with one's circumstances. This is thought to be the path to longevity, as well as the practices of living a simple life, caring for self and not eating too much, as expressed by a 68-year-old woman in Sydney (originally from Shanghai, Mainland China):

> I think in terms of simple lifestyle, natural food, sunlight and fresh air, and we should eat only until we are 70 per cent to 80 per cent full. We should relax and keep happy. People should live to one hundred year old. Good health should not depend on medicine. I think prevention is better than taking medicine.

The above expression reflects Taoist ideas for preserving health. Under this teaching, good health is maintained as much as possible with good eating habits, rather than by resorting to medicine once good health is lost. Sun Si-maio (Tang Dynasty) advised taking the right quantity of food at regular times: 'Eat when you are hungry, and drink when you are thirsty'. He also said, 'too full dinner at night will take away one's life' (Yiu 1984:180). In this quote from a 27-year-old woman in Sydney (originally from Hong Kong) is reflected the Taoist recommendation for 'simple food':

> Chinese elderly do not eat so many sweet foods. I think simple foods are good for health… My mother said the Traditional Chinese Medicines *huaishan* and *astragalus* are good for health.

This woman looked after elderly people in an aged care institution. One of the things that struck her most about the eating habits of the Western elderly was the considerable amount of sweet foods that were consumed, leading her to point out that this was not generally the way of the Chinese elderly.

For a 76-year-old woman in Sydney (originally from Mainland China), the meaning of Traditional Chinese Medicine soup also linked with the philosophies of simplicity, contentment, and adherence to nature advocated by Tao:

> I have enough to eat. I do not buy good food to eat or anything to nourish my body. I eat mostly vegetables. I do not feel like eating meat. Now, I stick to Chinese vegetables. I prefer to steam and boil chicken. I use chicken thighs to boil soups and add some Traditional Chinese Medicine, such as *Yu Zhu* (玉竹), the so-called dried assorted vegetables.

This woman had endured considerable hardship during thirty years of her life. She was born in a poor family in Mainland China. During the Japanese invasion she was kidnapped and sold to people in an isolated place. Most often she did not have enough food to eat. She gave birth to a baby boy, but he did not survive because of poverty and lack of medical facilities. She came to Australia after the death of her husband. In spite of her tragic past and poor living conditions, she had been happily settled and living in Australia for more than fourteen years. She admitted that even though in the past she had been hungry when she had no food, now that food was abundant she could not (or dared not) eat too much. She adhered to a simple food regime by eating more vegetables and less meat, and steaming and boiling the meat that she did eat. Chicken thighs were less fattening according to her, and she used them for preparing Traditional Chinese Medicine soup.

Vegetables and mild Traditional Chinese Medicine soup are considered healthy, simple foods. In *Tao Te Ching* (chapter 53) simple food with little taste is recommended:

> Do that which consists of taking no action; pursue that which is not meddlesome; savour that which has no flavour.

Lau Tzu thought no flavour ranked highest among all flavours in food. This notion established a special aesthetic view and taste choice based on simplicity. For him, too much taste would be injurious, as expressed in *Tao Te Ching* (chapter 12): 'the five tastes injure his palate'. Foods with thick flavours which were produced by brewing and blending were believed to be toxic and to cause illness (Zhu 1994, cited in Flaws 1994).

Traditional Chinese Medicine and longevity

In the relationship between Traditional Chinese Medicine and longevity arise the concepts of using Traditional Chinese Medicine to nourish *qi* and the importance of its use in conjunction with exercise. A 50-year-old woman in Sydney (originally from Hong Kong) linked longevity in people she had known with their use of Traditional Chinese Medicine:

> People say that ginseng is for longevity – that ginseng can prolong your life and nourish *qi*. My husband's grandmother and grandfather used to eat lots of ginseng soup. His grandfather died at the age of ninety-six, and his grandmother is now around ninety-six or ninety-eight.

Moreover, she believed that eating nourishing Traditional Chinese Medicine such as ginseng provides energy; since energy is a sign of good health, having energy foods can prolong life. *Qi*, as articulated by this woman, is a vital concept in Traditional Chinese Medicine; it is defined as the force that binds all life (including heaven, earth and humans). It is also seen to be supplied in food. This association between *qi* and food can even be identified in the calligraphy. The character for *qi* 氣 is made up of two parts, the top part indicating 'rising vapour' and the lower part meaning 'rice'. Thus *qi* literally means 'vapour rising from rice' (Unschuld 1985:72).

The next statement reveals how a 70-year-old woman in Sydney (originally from Mainland China) shared this belief in the importance of eating nourishing Traditional Chinese Medicine for prolonging life. She felt the secret of her mother's longevity was eating well and taking Traditional Chinese Medicine:

> My mother had a long life. She died at the age of 98. She did not have many health problems. She walked well, ate well, and had black hair. Apart from exercise, my father bought her lots of deer antler. She took lots of that, and she was seldom ill.

We notice that these women in Sydney (the 50-year-old originally from Hong Kong and the 70-year-old originally from Mainland China) speak of 'eating more' Traditional Chinese Medicine, which appears to contrast with the views expressed by another two women in Sydney (both originally from Mainland China, one 76 years old and the other 68 years old) and the Brisbane group (originally from Taiwan), who suggested that eating too much is not good. These metaphors of 'more is better' or 'less is better', in relation to size, are deeply grounded in culture (Lakoff & Johnson 1980). In traditional Chinese societies, having plentiful food, especially expensive foods, was socially significant. Plentiful and expensive foods symbolised 'prosperity' and 'social status'. Social convention attached more importance to being 'plump' especially for girls and women, as being fatter was considered ideal for reproduction. Fat children were considered to be a sign of wealth as well as health. In contrast, in modern societies such as Hong Kong and Taiwan, the slogan now is 'the slimmer the better' and fat people have become stigmatised.

The theme linking Traditional Chinese Medicine and longevity with 'exercise' was discussed by a 50-year-old man in Armidale, (originally from Taiwan) and a 62-year-old man in Sydney (originally from See Yup, Mainland China). Both pointed out the importance of exercise for enhancing the effects of Traditional Chinese Medicine for longevity:

> Traditional Chinese Medicine can only benefit longevity when taken into account with exercise. Medicine alone will not work. I do not think I am doing well to achieve longevity because of the lack of exercise.

> If your health is good, you will have a long life. Taking Traditional Chinese Medicine can prolong your life. Of course some Traditional Chinese Medicine can regulate *yin* and *yang*, that is, regulate our bodies. Added to this is exercise, which will enhance longevity.

In traditional Chinese medical terms, exercise is said to enhance the circulation of *qi* and blood, strengthen the function of the spleen and stomach, and increase the body's immunity to disease (Flaws 1994:69). Chinese experts on longevity advised avoiding excessive comfort as this would impair health, yet exercise was also to be well-balanced and moderate according to Sun Si-miao (quoted by Sun 1988:142, in Flaws 1994:71): 'The body desires labour, but one should never labour to extremes'.

Traditional Chinese Medicine and fatalism

However, some participants also expressed disbelief in the association between Traditional Chinese Medicine and longevity. These people viewed life as being predetermined, and they held a fatalistic belief that human efforts have no influence over how long one lives. This idea can be referenced to Wong Chung (王充) (CE 27 – ca.100), a philosopher during the Han period, who put forward the idea that fate governs life:

> The good fortune or harm encountered by man all comes from Fate. There is a Fate governing death and life, long or short existence, and also Fate governing riches and honours, poverty and [low] position.

> (Fung 1973:164)

Individual's perceptions on this matter will be influenced by philosophy as well as by personal life experiences. A 74-year-old woman in Sydney (originally from See Yup, Mainland China) had this view:

> Eating Traditional Chinese Medicine for longevity? Impossible, life is predestined. I have had life enough.

This woman's fatalistic view stemmed from her life experiences. She had endured many hardships as a woman during times of war and poverty in China. She felt her life experiences had been predestined and that she had no reason to look forward to a better life. To some Chinese people, fate is considered in the contexts of time and place – whether one is born at the right time (peaceful) and at the right place (wealthy family). Mencius (*Kung-sun Chau*, part 2) proposed that these three elements are important aspects of human encounters: the opportunities of time, advantages of situation, and harmony with people (天時地利人和). Note the first two of these are determined by fate.

In contrast, the 77-year-old man in Sydney (originally from Shanghai, Mainland China) presented a different picture as one who was born 'with a golden key in the mouth', with good fortune. Most of his life he had had a comfortable and easy life, with little reason for worry. Born into a wealthy and caring family, he had all the material comforts and support he needed when he was young, and did not feel the need to seek out additional safeguards:

> I do not believe that Traditional Chinese Medicine helps longevity, but my wife does, and she will prepare me some ginseng tea occasionally. I would not do it myself. According to my own experience, I have never tried to look for something.

Our body, according to the following remarks from the 80-year-old man in Brisbane (originally from Hong Kong) was like a motor car that would eventually wear-out, and thus death was inevitable. He admitted he had a good life and was ready to go at anytime. He had what most people wish for: fame, money and power. However he was depressed when he recounted the story of how his Australian wife had died unexpectedly. Lonely years were stretching ahead for him and there was nothing left for him to anticipate. He said that human lives were unpredictable and that ill fortune could happen anytime:

> I do not believe that Traditional Chinese Medicine can help longevity. Once you are over 60, your life is on standby, just like waiting to catch the plane. Your body is just like the motor car you drive all day and all night. It must go bad somewhere, sometime. How can you get new parts?

Reflections

The conviction that good health and human relationships can be achieved through personal efficacy and health strategies underlies the pursuit of Traditional Chinese Medicine by some of these participants. These strategies are implemented to fulfil various social obligations in three key stages of life: youth, adulthood, and old age. Traditional Chinese Medicine in youth focuses on building vitality, with Traditional Chinese Medicine playing a preventive role and laying the foundation for the destinies of masculinity and reproduction. For adult males, the special emphasis in Traditional Chinese Medicine is on maximising virility, through which sexuality and manhood are affirmed. For adult females, Traditional Chinese Medicine is focused on the priorities of enhancing fertility and obtaining healthy children. For the elderly, preserving health by adhering to health regimes is seen as critical for healthy aging. Traditional Chinese Medicine is related to successful ageing and longevity in conjunction with exercise, and Traditional Chinese Medicine as food is used in the belief that it will nourish *qi*.

This chapter elaborates on two key concepts. Firstly, it is believed that vitality in health and human relationships can be achieved by pursuing a health regime based on the precepts of Traditional Chinese Medicine, in terms of dietary advice and life practices. Significantly, we have uncovered symbolic aspects of the consumption of Traditional Chinese Medicine in participants' health beliefs. Assimilating powerful animals symbolises exhibiting power through conquest. Concepts of both 'eating more' or 'eating less' in healthy living and of being born at the right time and in the right place have been associated with longevity. Secondly, vigour and virility encompass social meanings with regard to family obligations and continuing the family line, a combination of cultural beliefs and social practices. Gender and sexual biases throughout Chinese cultural history are still apparent in the gendered use of Traditional Chinese Medicine.

Pursuing a balanced healthy life and personal efficacy with the utmost vigour, in line with traditional cultural beliefs and social practices, reveal the importance of ensuring the continuation of the family line as well as a productive personal future.

These social discourses in Traditional Chinese Medicine are further explored in the discourses of 'family connectedness' in the next chapter, which throws further light on the social expectations surrounding the administration and practice of Traditional Chinese Medicine.

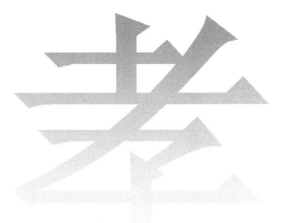

chapter six

Family Connectedness

(Pronounced as *haau*, which means 'filial piety')

Traditional Chinese Medicine has linked us together since I was a child. It is often used in a family context.

A 45-year-old man in Armidale
(from Beijing, Mainland China)

Introduction

Traditional Chinese Medicine as family connectedness embodies the profound meaning of filial piety, a crucial element in Chinese culture. Filial piety defines harmonious relationships by mutual obligation within a family, extending outside to friends. Significantly, Traditional Chinese Medicine is a vehicle for the transmission and continuation of culture, both in its use for the continuity of family lines and by its linking of generations through tradition.

This chapter is concerned with the practices and underlying symbolic meanings employed by participants in implementing this continuation of culture.

The practices include the maternal bond, children's respect manifested in the non-material sense, carrying on ancient cultural practices and traditions, and sharing with friends.

In this chapter, the Chinese concept of honouring the past, the foundation of filial piety, is explored, followed by the Chinese family system and its role, and concepts of filial piety. Contrasting cases documenting discontinuity are included, providing a complementary perspective from which to view varied social realities.

Honouring the past

For many Chinese people, honouring the past has profound cultural significance. Many people have been imbued with the thinking that 'ever lasting' is as long as history. This way of thinking dates back to the Warring States Period (475–221 BCE), when the idea of clinging to the past was expounded in *The Doctrine of the Mean* (400–500 BCE) as a way to honour past ancestors, an extension of filial piety:

> Filial piety is seen in the skilful carrying out the wishes of our forefathers, and the skilful carrying forward of their undertakings.

> (*The Doctrine of the Mean*, chapter 19, section 1)

Examples abound in *The Doctrine of the Mean* of Chinese emperors of the past respecting their ancestors (chapter 19, section 5):

> They revered those whom they honoured, and loved those whom they regarded with affection. Thus they served the dead as they would have served them alive; they served the departed as they would have served them had they been continued among them 事死人如事生, 事亡如事存.

Continuity with the past is amply implied in the statement, 'Reaching far and continuing long, this is how it perfects all things' (*The Doctrine of the Mean*, chapter 26, section 4). Lao Tzu (600–400 BCE) encouraged people to follow 'the ever lasting' heaven and earth.

Chinese people tend to glorify past experiences and history, remembering the dead and building memorials and temples as signs of respect (Lam & Wong 1995). The past is not 'gone'; it links up with the present and provides a basis for the future. This sentiment has been described as having certain elements of ancestor worship and infatuation (Leung 1995). Another suggestion is that traditional Chinese people are proud of the past, trust the wisdom of ancestors, and consider past teachings and family rules handed down as forever true (Wai 1995). Continuity with the past is based on 'trust', which is a basic virtue in Traditional Chinese culture (Qian 1993). Trust and reverence are important in the social contract. If one trusts and reveres the past, one will be trusted and revered in the future. This indicates the importance placed on reciprocal social relationships.

However, one important notion is continuity through change. Reality is understood as constantly changing and dynamic, and nothing is absolute, as expounded in *The Book of Changes* (Baynes 1965). This 'change' concept is fundamental to Traditional Chinese Medicine, where diagnosis is based on perceiving disease in terms of dynamic patterns which are always in a state of flux, for which harmony is the goal (Zhang & Rose 1999).

Continuity is a means of preservation, despite change. For example, Chinese people have always wanted to preserve something to pass on to future generations. Continuity and virtue is especially important. The ancient Chinese scholar Sse-ma Kwong (司馬光) explained (my translation):

> If you try to save money for future generations, they may not know how to safeguard it; if you want to keep books for future generations, they may not know how to read; the best way is to accumulate 'virtues' for the ever-lasting plan of future generations.

> (Wai 1995:29)

One way of accumulating virtues for following generations is to nurture a sound character. This emphasis on 'virtues' is a driving force in the continuity of Chinese culture. Indeed, as modern historian Qian (1993) has pointed out, there are two dimensions to Chinese culture: morality and arts. Confucius's teachings represent the moral dimension of Chinese culture and Taoism represents the artistic side. There is an ancient saying that 'virtue begins at home'. Let us now look at the Chinese family system, which governs the thoughts and action of many Chinese people and is largely influenced by Confucianism.

Chinese family system

Traditionally, Chinese social life centres on the family. Mencius suggests that the family is the basis of a country (Lau 1978). The social ideal for every member of the family is to know one's role and to adhere to expected social obligations. These are defined in the five cardinal human relationships: ruler and follower, father and son, husband and wife, older and younger brothers, and friends. As modern historian Fung Yu-lan (Leung 1994) pointed out, three out of the five categories are directly related to family, namely, the relationship between father and son, husband and wife, older brother and younger brother. Moreover, the remaining two are indirectly related to familial relationships in the way Chinese people often address the ruler as 'father' and friends as 'brothers'. The drawback of this family consciousness, as Lin (1977:164) argued, was a degeneration into a state of 'magnified selfishness'. It was argued that under this system a walled castle was created separating the family inside from the outside world; social obligations toward strangers received less emphasis and the Samaritan virtue was given little credence. However, theoretically public spirit was implicit in the ideas of reciprocity. Helping others was configured as a way of helping oneself: 'Wanting to be successful himself, he helps others to be successful; wanting to stand on his own feet, he helps others to stand on their feet' (Lin 1977:172). However, these 'others' were not clearly defined in terms of the cardinal relationships.

Role of the family

A prime function of the family was social, cultural and biological reproduction – the survival of the family line. This was also Confucius's (551–479 BCE) main concern:

> The old shall be made to live in peace and security, the young shall learn to love and be loyal, that inside the chamber, there may be no unmarried maids, and outside the chamber there may be no unmarried males.

> (Lin 1938:196)

Biological aspects of life can be further seen in the arrangement of life within a family structure: giving birth in a family, growing old in a family, becoming sick in the family, and dying in a family. From a health care point of view, family took the role that hospitals take in modern times; family provided care for the sick, and family members were the nurses. When someone died, family members attended to the burial (Leung 1994). In this way, family provided a means of social survival and family continuity throughout the cycle of life and death.

Another function of the family was transmission of culture and tradition. Malinowski (1963:39) asserted that family was the social means for continuity of traditions. He argued that in many societies, as in China in ancient days, to have many children was perceived to be 'economically advantageous, morally desirable and socially honourable'. This is understandable as children provided help both inside a family and as agricultural labour in traditional Chinese societies. Children, especially sons, were considered important for safeguarding old age, and for the reciprocal pride of having children. The core Confucian value of 'filial piety' established the system of obligation that ensured the stability and continuation of this Chinese cultural structure based on family.

Filial piety

Chinese people generally consider filial piety to be pre-eminent among the hundreds of moral principles. Filial piety is a code of social conduct governing human relationships, and its meaning and purpose are clearly defined in the following statements:

> Filial piety is the foundation of all virtues and the fountainhead where all moral teaching springs... Filial piety begins with the service of our parents, proceeds to serve the emperor and is consummated in establishing ourselves in the world and achieving attainments.

> (*Classic of Filial Piety* 722 CE:29)

The basis of filial piety is the reciprocal relationship between parents and children in traditional Chinese families – parents try their best to look after their children and children in return show respect to their parents. The Chinese character for filial piety (孝) consists of two parts – the top part refers to 'the elderly', the lower part means 'son'. The meaning derives from the idea of the son supporting the elderly, and the elderly being above the son. Moreover, 'reverence' is a virtue which distinguishes humans from animals. This principle is stated in the *Analects*:

> Filial piety means the support of one's parents. But dogs and horses likewise are able to do something in the way of support; without reverence, what is there to distinguish the one support given from the other?

> (*Analects*, Book 2, chapter 7)

Filial piety is sustained by serving parents while they are alive and by proper burial when they are dead, as seen in the following passage.

Those parents, when alive, should be served according to propriety; that when dead, they should be buried according to propriety;

(*Analects*, Book 2, chapter 2)

According to historian Qian (1993), filial piety is a responsibility, because the virtues of filial piety already reside in oneself; all one needs to do is act accordingly. Someone who shows complete filial piety can be said to have acquired the 'twenty-four examples of filial piety' (二十四孝), a popular saying among Chinese people.

Maternal bond

A common Chinese saying is that 'a woman's place is at home'. Home is considered the very place where a woman can find her honourable self-expression, especially when a woman becomes a mother. A mother makes social continuity through the family line possible by her contribution to reproduction and caring for offspring. Some participants in the present study favourably recall the assiduous attention and tender loving care of their mothers who nurtured them while they were children, often expressed through the use of Traditional Chinese Medicine. In the participants' eyes, their mothers were models of perfection – gentle, loving, and self-sacrificing; above all, their mothers constantly supported them in times of good health and illness. The preparation and use of Traditional Chinese Medicine was commonly seen by participants as a symbol of maternal love in caring for a sick child, keeping herself healthy and independent so as not to be a burden to sons, and expressing care by preparing complicated Traditional Chinese Medicine, and in metaphors such as putting the mother's heart into preparing Traditional Chinese Medicine soups for children.

Preparing Traditional Chinese Medicine is all I can do

When thinking about her experience of Traditional Chinese Medicine, the first thing that came to the mind of a 70-year-old woman in Sydney (originally from Mainland China) was the care her own mother gave her when she was young, when her mother would say:

I know you are in pain. If you are overloaded, I can help you to shoulder the weight, but not when you are unwell. All I can do is to prepare you some herbal tea.

The mother indicated her psychological support, and used Traditional Chinese Medicine as the vehicle for helping her daughter. These caring and understanding words were spoken against a background of poverty in a village in Mainland China where Western medicine was unavailable and Chinese herbs were the most economical means available for treating illness. In this participant's childhood experience, it was a traditional practice for her mother to collect herbs in the mountains and prepare herbs for the family when they were ill.

That parents try their best to care for their children when they are sick is also evident in Confucius's teachings, in which caring for the young was emphasised:

> Mang Wu asked what filial piety was. The Master said,
> Parents are anxious lest their children should be sick.

> (*Analects*, Book 2, chapter 4)

Not a burden to sons

For the 80-year-old woman in Sydney (originally from See Yup, Mainland China), experience with Traditional Chinese Medicine reminded her of her wealthy past, when her mother was able to give her an expensive bird's nest to eat, but her thoughts also went to the period when she cared for her own son and was living in impoverished conditions. During the hardships of her life, she had struggled to survive whilst raising two sons on her own. She became careful about her food and learned to prepare Traditional Chinese Medicine soups in order to keep healthy. The reason she gave for using Traditional Chinese Medicine soups was to protect her sons:

> I am not afraid of anything, except that I do not want to be a burden to my son [who lived with her]. My sons are more important than my own life!

A mother's consideration for her sons is clearly expressed. The key word is 'burden'. She did not want to give her sons trouble by having to care for her if she became ill. She used Traditional Chinese Medicine to safeguard her health and to be independent. She considered her life insignificant when compared to the lives of her sons. Earlier in her life, her father, considering her lonely struggle, had suggested that she give the boys away and remarry, but she had not wanted to risk her sons going to bad people. She recalled a difficult time when she was hungry. Her reminiscences were punctuated with stories of her sacrifice and selfless love. As a considerate and devoted mother, it was not possible for her to eat alone in spite of her hunger:

> I got one bun and tried to eat, but I thought of my sons having nothing to eat, and I put the bun down.

'Chicken at five'

Another expression of maternal love through Traditional Chinese Medicine is found in an account of preparing complicated Traditional Chinese Medicine. A 70-year-old woman in Sydney (originally from Singapore) was brought up in a traditional family, and expressed her maternal devotion through Traditional Chinese Medicine by meticulously preparing bird's nest soup for her son. The so-called 'chicken at five' (五更雞) refers to a bird's nest prepared with chicken, which is ready for consumption at five in the morning.

The traditional preparation method was time-consuming and energy-demanding, involving a sequence of complicated steps: removing feathers from the bird's nest, putting the soup in her son's bedroom, checking the temperature of the soup, waking her son in the early morning and offering him the soup. She would then pass him a cup of water and a small pot for him to rinse his mouth after taking the sweet soup (which was prepared by adding rock sugar), and provided a small towel for him to wipe his mouth before he slept again. She believed that taking food at that time was ten times more beneficial than taking it during the day. Her rationale was that when one was sound asleep, one's lungs and stomach were opened and more absorptive. Importantly, there was no better way to express her care than by doing things herself:

> If you want those closest to you to get the benefit from eating, you must give your time and heart in preparing Traditional Chinese Medicine.

This vignette highlights the reasons why she employed such complicated steps for preparing Traditional Chinese Medicine for her son – by committing herself fully to giving her 'time' and her 'heart'.

Chicken soup with my heart in it

The giving of one's heart in preparing Traditional Chinese Medicine was echoed in many participants, such as this 58-year-old woman in Sydney (originally from Mainland China) who prepared soup with her 'heart' in it:

I prepare Traditional Chinese Medicine soup for my children. They drink my soup like having 'chicken soup with my heart in it' (人心雞湯).

This woman in Sydney expressed, metaphorically, the transcendent meaning of Traditional Chinese Medicine. Since the mother was 'good' to her children, the chicken soup that she prepared became a metaphor of soup made with her heart, symbolising her care and goodwill toward her children.

A mother needs 'three hearts and two attentions' (三心二意). Three hearts means a loving heart, a consistent heart, and a determined heart.

Here, she expands on her conception of being a good mother as requiring three hearts, loving, consistent and determined. However the original Chinese expression of 'three hearts and two attentions' has a different meaning, referring to people having too many ideas and having trouble deciding which is which. However, in the present context this metaphor prescribes three strategies for dealing with children, which require care, consistency and firmness.

Her maternal love was revealed on one occasion when her children were immersed in cold water for treatment. When she saw their hands and legs shaking, she cried out and grasped her children at once. Regardless of what other people said, she thought:

I feel pain to look at them exposed in such a way – they are my children, no matter whether they are my first child or my tenth one.

These feelings reflect Confucian teachings on caring for the young:

In regard to the young, treat them tenderly.

(*Analects*, Book 5, chapter 25:4)

The words of the four Chinese women whose quotes appear in this section illustrate mothers' selfless devotion to their children. These women believed it was important to give of their time and hearts to attend to their children. They struggled hard in life, even forgetting their own pain in their preference for caring for their children. They all came from traditional Chinese societies and had learned the reciprocal values of filial piety.

Children were considered important in the traditional patriarchal family, especially in agricultural societies, for looking after the land and safeguarding the elderly. Sun Yat-sen (1963) suggested that children living under the patriarchal family system had more protection and security than in the modern family, where children are allowed to have more freedom.

Reciprocity, a characteristic of the traditional Chinese family, involved a bond between fathers and sons (Wai 1995). When sons were young, fathers tried their best to provide for them, so that one day they would be well looked after in return. Gouldner (Larson 1977:163), in his social exchange theory, stated that the norm of reciprocity is a universal cultural phenomenon, and that reciprocity creates social stability as a result of mutual social indebtedness.

However, filial piety could also be viewed as a form of social control under which people have narrowly defined roles and are expected to reciprocate. It involved an unconditional self-renunciation of one's independence, and it was through the sons' respect for their fathers that they realised their own roles. It has been argued that filial piety originated as a means of governing people. The assumption was that if everyone conformed to filial piety, no one would dare to rebel against the rulers and peace would prevail (Lau 1978). This is particularly the case when the emperor is to be considered as a father figure.

Often mothers' relationships with their children have been closer than fathers', which could be more distant relationships. A review of the literature reveals that continuity with sex-role differentiation remains; that is, mother–child relations are more affective and closer in modern Chinese societies than father–child relationships (Ho 1989). The *Book of Rites* or *Li Ki* (quoted in Dawson 1995:52), a Confucian canon, sets out the regulations for the family. Regarding parent–child relationships it says:

> The mother deals with them on grounds of affection rather than pride, and the father on grounds of pride rather than affection.

> (*Li Ki*, Book 29:29)

Moreover, the expression of parental care often occurs not so much in parents' words to their children, but coded into their actions. According to Confucius's teaching, action and words must be matched:

> The reason why the ancients did not readily give utterance to their words was that they feared lest their actions should not come up to them.

> (*Analects*, Book 5, chapter 22)

This expression of care in action but not in words was illustrated by a 77-year-old man in Sydney (originally from Shanghai, Mainland China):

My parents' concern to me was expressed in the way that they asked me to eat more, including Traditional Chinese Medicine. My mother might love me a great deal, but she would not say so. It was their 'virtue' not to show their feelings.

This man had been able to access all forms of Traditional Chinese Medicine when he was in China because of his family's high status and social position. His parents gave him plenty of good foods, including expensive Traditional Chinese Medicine. Note the reserved expression of love by his parents, especially his mother, shown in action but not in words; this was a social norm and considered a virtue in his parents' traditional society.

Children's reciprocal return

In the previous section, we saw mothers ensuring the survival of family lines through material expressions of maternal love toward their children, in this case exemplified by their use of Traditional Chinese Medicine. In this section, the survival and continuity of culture and family lines are further guaranteed by their children. Parental affection toward children is seen to be natural, yet the reciprocation of children's affection toward parents needs to be cultivated. As suggested by Lin (1938:198), 'a natural man loves his children, but a cultured man loves his parents'. Filial piety, children's sense of obligation and gratitude toward their parents, is codified in the works of Mencius who said that children should not only show joy but should always remember:

When one is loved by one's parents, though pleased, one must not forget.

(*Wan Zhang*, part A, chapter 5, trans. Lau 1970:138)

Of all my duties, which is the greatest? My duty to my own parents!

(*Li Lou*, part A, chapter 4, trans. Lau 1970:125)

The first statement speaks of dual feelings toward parents, of feeling happy for having loving parents, and of being grateful and reciprocating when one is capable. The second statement positions the reciprocal obligation of children toward their parents as the children's greatest duty.

A sense of gratitude towards parents was demonstrated in two ways by some younger participants in this study; intangibly, by offering care and showing respect, and tangibly through material returns.

Saying thank you and taking action

The experience of Traditional Chinese Medicine for a 21-year-old man in Brisbane (originally from Hong Kong) was gratitude and sincere promise:

> I had bird's nest every day when my skin was bad. I have to thank my parents. I tell them all the time that I would take care of them.

Significantly, he embraced his duty to look after his parents because of his experience with Traditional Chinese Medicine. Again the emphasis is on 'doing': for many Chinese people there is no point in speaking without action. As stated by Confucius in the previous section, speech should be congruent with action. The action, in terms of returning favours to parents, acknowledges the traditional Chinese idea of obligation. Again, the young man showed the reciprocal nature of obligation:

> Whose mother does not want to be looked after by her son? Who else has the time to give birth to a son?

The first question he raises perhaps does not have an automatic answer in this modern society. The second question is striking, using the busy lives of women as a counterpoint, and considering the changing role of mothers in modern Chinese societies such as Hong Kong. Many women undertake a double role of working outside the family as well as taking care of children, though many domestic tasks can be alleviated by employing foreign domestic servants. Because of the double role of women in Hong Kong, the young man appreciated his mother more for finding time to care for him.

Kneeling and offering a cup of tea

In the next case, acts of filial piety are illustrated by the traditional Chinese custom of kneeling and offering a cup of tea during Chinese New Year. A 27-year-old woman in Sydney (originally from Hong Kong), had rhinitis, headache and skin allergy. Her mother suggested she consult an acupuncturist and use Traditional Chinese Medicine. She listened to her mother and tried various Traditional Chinese Medicine modalities as instructed, conforming with the demands of filial piety. She acknowledges she is reserved and traditional:

> On Chinese New Year, I would kneel and offer my mother a cup of tea. That is very traditional. I think it is right to show filial piety since my mother gave birth to me. I try to keep this tradition.

Chinese New Year is an occasion for families to gather together and to pay their respects to parents or seniors in the family. The traditional way for children to show their respect to their parents is to kneel and offer them a cup of tea. In return, the children would get *lai-see* (利事), red envelopes with money inside, as a sign of blessing from their parents. This woman continued to learn Traditional Chinese Medicine mostly from her mother, who had considerable experience with Traditional Chinese Medicine foods; she said her mother was like a 'tape recorder', always talking about what she should and should not eat, day and night.

Feeling honourable and noble

Though the 30-year-old woman in Brisbane (originally from Papua New Guinea) was brought up in the mixed culture of Papua New Guinea, she had an affinity towards Chinese ways and understood the ethos of filial piety. One of the main influences behind her interest in Traditional Chinese Medicine had been her parents. Her father, whom she admired, was interested in Traditional Chinese Medicine. She credited her parents for the way they brought her up:

> I feel I am important as a person, and my mother treats me so that I feel important as a person. They do not give me pressure. If I want to do anything, they are very supportive.

She is considered an individual in her own right by her parents, and is given autonomy and support for her decisions. In that sense she has freedom at home, and experiences a modern style of living without pressure from parents. When she touched on the issue of looking after her parents, without hesitation she said this was an honourable and noble role for her to fulfil one day. The reciprocal nature of this relationship can be seen in her remarks:

> I feel an obligation; it is something that I do willingly, something that I feel is honourable and noble.

Material return

Two participants, originally from Hong Kong, fulfilled their obligations of filial piety by contributing money to their parents. Expressing gratitude by giving money to parents is socially acceptable in Hong Kong (King 1996). In the mix of Chinese and Western culture that is Hong Kong, material expression is part of people's social lives. Even Weber (1951:242) was aware of the 'crass materialism' of the Chinese! Of course, the symbolic meaning of showing respect in terms of material return is important. The reciprocal relationship in giving and taking is clear in the following accounts.

A 56-year-old woman in Armidale (originally from Hong Kong), said that her mother used to prepare different types of Traditional Chinese Medicine for her when she was young, ranging from simple herbal teas to health tonics. Moreover, her mother's lively social spirit, and her rich knowledge of Traditional Chinese Medicine were what she remembered and learned from most. When she was independent and started working, she adhered to the traditional Chinese custom of giving money to her mother as a sign of filial piety:

> When I was a child and had fever, my mother gave me 'seven star tea.' When I had too much fried foods, she gave me 'five flowers tea'. When I started my period, I had *dong quan*. I went home and gave money to my mother, and kept a very small amount for myself.

This 50-year-old woman in Sydney (originally from Hong Kong) spoke of reciprocal return in terms of money:

> My mother is a traditional thinker. She used Traditional Chinese Medicine for soup. She would prepare pork heart with Traditional Chinese Medicine for me when I had examinations. The purpose was to calm my examination fears. I have a strong adherence to family tradition; I give money to my mother when I get paid and buy things for her.

We learn that her mother knew the traditional way to prepare Traditional Chinese Medicine and that certain foods were used with therapeutic intent. Chinese people believe that eating heart will nourish their inner strength. This woman also expressed her attachment to the family tradition of giving money to her mother. She had been exposed to Chinese culture during her studies in Chinese middle school, and was very much influenced by her teachers. To give money to her mother was a natural way to behave.

Family as knowledge transmission

Parents transmit traditional cultural knowledge to their children as they educate them to establish 'sound' characters and to contribute to society (Wai 1995). One fine example was given by a 48-year-old woman in Sydney (originally from Hong Kong), whose experience of learning about Traditional Chinese Medicine from her mother can be divided into three phases: sharing, separation, and continuity.

Sharing. She recalled sharing the experience of Traditional Chinese Medicine as a child with her mother in terms of seeing, learning and tasting. She said that as a child, 'health was the best gift from my mother'.

Separation. When this woman was six years old, her mother's health started to deteriorate. Her mother was diagnosed with cancer, and tried various types of Traditional Chinese Medicine. While her mother was ill, the woman's experience changed from sharing to being the one responsible for preparing the Traditional Chinese Medicine for her mother. Eventually her mother died when she was twelve years old, leaving her with the heavy burden of caring for her younger brother and sister.

Continuity. She had a very unhappy marriage and decided to run away and lead a life of her own. One thing she took with her was her knowledge of Traditional Chinese Medicine that she had received from her mother:

> When I ran away from home, I carried my Traditional Chinese Medicine wine with me [which her mother had taught her to prepare].

In spite of the changes in her life, this one thing remained unchanged. Her mother's spirit lived on in her heart through her continued commitment to using Traditional Chinese Medicine knowledge, and in this way she honoured her mother's memory.

Interacting with friends

Friendships can enrich and complement the family learning experience, as reflected in Confucius's teaching:

> The superior man on literary grounds meets with his friends, and by their friendship helps his virtues.
>
> (*Analects*, Book 4, chapter 3)

Confucius's vision of benevolence includes filial piety, the extension of which is to treat all people in society as 'brothers', the ideal of 'one big family'. Accordingly, one's social life becomes contiguous with one's family. Traditional Chinese Medicine also provides a means for social interaction with friends, and this is represented in the following accounts.

For a 70-year-old woman in Sydney (originally from Singapore), she was able to continue her social life through Traditional Chinese Medicine, a process which she experienced through two phases: self-esteem and social continuity.

Self-esteem. She said: 'I did not accept myself too well'. She was very conscious of her appearance from the time she was a teenager, and described herself as tall and skinny with a big head, like 'a doll'. This metaphor denotes a sense of unreality in her sense of self. However her body image changed over time. Her figure, which she once rejected as being too thin, is now considered fashionable. In Hong Kong, a contemporary saying is 'the slimmer the better' (echoed by a 40-year-old woman in Armidale, originally from Hong Kong). This differs from earlier times, when being plump was considered to indicate health and wealth, and was more socially desirable.

Social continuity. Sharing Traditional Chinese Medicine was a means for her to regain her spirit; she gave Traditional Chinese Medicine to her friends and their children, though she consumed very little herself:

> I had a sharing spirit; I did not just care for those people near me, but also for my friends and their children, and I was willing to give them Traditional Chinese Medicine to try.

The above discourses illustrate the status of Traditional Chinese Medicine as a worthy gift and as symbolising a caring spirit expressed through sharing, first with her family and then to friends and their children. Moreover, this woman in Sydney followed the traditional methods for preparing Traditional Chinese Medicine and also shared her knowledge with her friends. This socially-connected spirit can be explained through Mencius's moral doctrine of *yen* or benevolence, the highest standard for one's living. Benevolence is part of human nature, according to the works of Mencius; benevolence should originate within the family and then be extended to the outside world:

> He who feels the love of family towards his own kin will feel humanity for all men. He who feels humanity for all men will be kind to all living creatures.

> (*Mencius*, trans. Dobson 1963:139)

According to principle of *yen*, benevolence is a universal love which starts at home and extends to all. Benevolence is an extension of kindness that implies expansion into social action – 'a heart that cannot bear the suffering of others'. The expression of benevolence is given in the example of 'a child about to fall into a well' (*Kung-sun Chau*, part 1, chapter 6, section 3), an event that would alarm us and move us to compassion. Compassion is the foundation of benevolence. Thus the progression from serving parents to concern and caring for people and things outside the family – that is, from familial love to universal love – is considered a true expression of benevolence. Traditional Chinese Medicine is an important vehicle for realising these idealistic principles.

The actions of an 80-year-old man in Sydney (originally from Mainland China) also exemplified the sharing spirit implied in using Traditional Chinese Medicine as a valuable gift. His continuing practice of using Traditional Chinese Medicine and sharing it with his friends mirrored his past experience. When he was a child, his mother prepared Traditional Chinese Medicine for the whole family from herbs she collected in the nearby mountains. He also learned from his school teacher how to make use of scarce resources. After he came to Australia he was much attracted by Australia's flowers and plants, and he continued the ways of his mother and his teacher. He planted many Traditional Chinese Medicine herbs and shared them with his friends. He said that if one has knowledge of herbs, 'the mountain becomes a treasure, otherwise the whole mountain turns into grass' (滿山是寶, 滿山是草).

Another experience of Traditional Chinese Medicine representing social integration was related by a 21-year-old man in Brisbane (originally from Hong Kong). He described himself as having a 'very hot' body type, for which the cure was to use the cool type of medicine for balance. He had recently experienced severe dermatitis, including on his face:

> In these two years I have had severe dermatitis. I have been taking Traditional Chinese Medicine herbal teas in these two years.

His two years of Traditional Chinese Medicine experience reflected four themes: stigmatisation, social isolation, frustration and social reintegration.

Stigmatisation. His problem was so severe – 'my face was covered in weeping sores' – that he lost all his self confidence. In Hong Kong society, outward appearance is valued. He dared not see people and said he could not look at himself in the mirror.

Social isolation. He described himself as being 'imprisoned' during those two years. He seldom went out, apart from going to school, and he focused mainly on his studies. He believed that once he got good qualifications everything would fit in nicely, including love.

Frustration. He felt his body was not under his control, and he was frustrated that he was taking Western medicine which did not seem to be able to control his problem. He was prevented from doing what he wanted to do and it was affecting his social life.

Social reintegration. Once his appearance improved, apparently due to the effects of Traditional Chinese Medicine, he started to expand his activities from being at home to venturing into the outside world: 'I restarted my life again. I began to have a social life and make new friends'.

As family tradition

Tradition underwrites human interactions in particular societies; though traditions can evolve, the core values tend to be resilient. Shih (1981:12) contends that tradition is created through 'human actions, through thought and imagination. It is handed down from one generation to the next'. The continuity of our traditions and our past was evident in sociologist David Riesman's *The Lonely Crowd* (1963) in which he maintained that human behaviour is greatly influenced by traditions, the customs and rules passed down from previous generations and ancestors (Wai 1995).

Remembering the past recreates our sense of continuity. When a tradition is enacted, it becomes 'vivid' and 'vital' to the people who accept it as part of 'their action'. The present and the past are fused (Shils 1981). In this chapter, the reminiscences of people from a range of origins – Hong Kong, China, Taiwan and Papua New Guinea – illustrate the integral role that Traditional Chinese Medicine played in their experience of the continuity (or discontinuity) of family traditions.

Traditional Chinese Medicine in the form of foods shared among family members provides a social bond that unites people: it becomes part of the participants. Soups in particular are popular among Chinese people. Factors such as the length of the preparation time and the ingredients tend to be characteristic of regions. For example, soups prepared in the Canton area of China and Hong Kong and by Papua New Guinea Chinese people with origins in southern China are traditionally boiled for a prolonged period (around three hours for Traditional Chinese Medicine soups), whereas soup from Taiwan and Northern China has a much shorter preparation time.

In some families the tradition of sharing Traditional Chinese Medicine is so strong, it tends to be taken for granted, as articulated by this 69-year-old man in Brisbane (originally from Papua New Guinea):

I think lots of Chinese people take Traditional Chinese Medicine because it is handed down from their families; they do not ask whether it is effective or not, they just use it.

Traditional Chinese Medicine, a vital part of Chinese heritage, has been 'handed down' through a medical history of several thousand years. Discourses in Traditional Chinese Medicine symbolise survival and connection with the past. As suggested earlier, though Chinese people are receptive to Western ideas, they continue to adhere to ancient traditions (Zhang & Rose 1999).

This man's comments also speak of Traditional Chinese Medicine being taken as an act of faith, with people using it without needing to be freshly convinced of its effectiveness. This phenomenon can be attributed, in part, to a significant difference between modern Western and Chinese culture. This is the lack of an 'Enlightenment' era or application of scientific thought (in the modern sense) in the Chinese way of thinking (Wai 1995). As such, Chinese culture tends toward affection, morals and intuitive thinking, with an emphasis on subjective thinking and experience. Traditional Chinese Medicine is a more like a philosophical approach, a tradition and a set of beliefs, than Western medicine.

Ancient Chinese philosophical writings are replete with moral teachings, the basis of Chinese culture. Confucianism's moral teachings of 'filial piety', 'benevolence', 'righteousness' and 'loyalty' were developed as early as the Zhou Dynasty (1027–221 BCE) and continued to be influential in later dynasties. The 'Doctrine of Universal Love' put forward by Mohists was based on morality. This moral focus also permeated the teachings of Taoism, in concepts such as the unity of human and nature, non-action, and simplicity. Qin (221–207 BCE) scholars modelled their considerations on Taoist principles. Han (206 BCE – 220 CE) scholars favoured Confucianism, and considered it to be the central teaching. The Sung period (960–1279 CE) witnessed the redevelopment of Confucianism, and philosophers of that time praised a mentality of discipline and high morality.

This affective nature of Chinese thinking can be identified in the use of Traditional Chinese Medicine as part of family tradition linking family together, and is revealed in many of the interviews.

Linking family together

In the experience of this 30-year-old woman in Brisbane (originally from Papua New Guinea), her experience was of sharing Traditional Chinese Medicine in her family:

> We had a tonic we rubbed on our muscles… Everyone that I knew always had that. We were in Papua New Guinea at that time… We always had ginseng and at dinner I was always having soups for this and soups for that. My grandfather and my grandmother used to know a lot and passed it down.

Though she largely grew up in Brisbane, her early family tradition had a deep impact on her. Her grandfather was an herbalist, and her grandmother was knowledgeable about Traditional Chinese Medicine. Her father was also interested in Traditional Chinese Medicine. Traditional Chinese Medicine had become an integral part of her life. To her, 'Traditional Chinese Medicine is mainly about food', and she was very careful about what she ate. Her practice of good eating was practical evidence of the continuity of her family traditions and of the close association of food and medicine in Chinese culture.

In the case of a 71-year-old man, also living in Brisbane but who had earlier lived in Papua New Guinea, Traditional Chinese Medicine soup was an essential. His family, originally from See Yup, China, had continued to use Traditional Chinese Medicine soup:

> Of course Traditional Chinese Medicine soup is a must and very popular. You can get those soups from the shops in Papua New Guinea or in the shops around here [Brisbane].

The use of Traditional Chinese Medicine was strong in the culture of his family. His grandfather came from a village in China and knew Traditional Chinese Medicine, and his mother also shared Traditional Chinese Medicine with the family. He considered himself fortunate to have had contact with people who had recently come from China while he was in Papua New Guinea:

> I was lucky because there were Chinese there who came from China. We had interactions with Chinese people. We were able to try Traditional Chinese Medicine at least.

In this way, the use of Traditional Chinese Medicine was carried to quite remote and culturally varied settings. The Brisbane participants who were originally from Papua New Guinea spoke of their experience growing up with both Chinese and Western influences. Mixed businesses in Papua New Guinea sold Traditional Chinese Medicine ingredients. Chinese people used both Traditional Chinese Medicine and Western medicines (but mainly Western medicines), possibly in an attempt to get the best of both worlds.

In the experience of a 45-year-old man in Armidale (originally from Beijing, Mainland China), Traditional Chinese Medicine was a link to childhood and tradition:

> Traditional Chinese Medicine has linked us together since I was a child. It is often used in a family context.

The man in Armidale learnt Traditional Chinese Medicine at home mainly through its use with food and particularly from his mother, who prepared Traditional Chinese Medicine soup to strengthen him. Later he was inspired by reading *Dream of the Red Chamber*, a traditional Chinese classic novel at the Qing Dynasty (1644 –1911 CE) written by Tsao Hsueh-chin (c. 1717–1763, trans. Wang 1983). In one example of Traditional Chinese Medicine from the novel, a physician was consulted, made a diagnosis, and prescribed 'ginger'. On another occasion, a tonic made up of Traditional Chinese Medicine remedies such as cinnamon, aconitum seeds, turtle shell and ginseng was used.

For a 77-year-old man in Sydney (originally from Shanghai, Mainland China), Traditional Chinese Medicine meant 'food supplement' in his family tradition:

> My uncle taught us to take Traditional Chinese Medicine as health supplements. My parents listened to him. I was given Traditional Chinese Medicine to keep me 'warm'.

Although his family used Western medicine because of their high social status, his parents often consulted his uncle, a practitioner of Traditional Chinese Medicine, regarding food supplements. This man continued to use Traditional Chinese Medicine and believed in its value as a food supplement; at the same time he had regular check-ups with Western doctors in Australia.

Traditional Chinese Medicine was a profession and a hobby for a 62-year-old man in Sydney (originally came from Mainland China). Traditional Chinese Medicine was a tradition in his family, and he was inspired to become a practitioner by his father, who was a famous martial arts practitioner. Prior to studying martial arts himself, he had been required to study Traditional

Chinese Medicine. The rationale for learning Traditional Chinese Medicine was that it was a skill that he could apply to caring for himself before taking care of others. He had been learning martial arts for over fifty years, and was still practicing. He incorporated exercise in his Traditional Chinese Medicine program because martial arts were considered to be part of 'the inheritance of Traditional Chinese Medicine'.

Linking generations

Traditional Chinese Medicine as part of the culture has been passed from generation to generation, sustaining the traditions of Traditional Chinese Medicine. A 50-year-old man in Armidale had a favourable recollection of Traditional Chinese Medicine from his youth in Taiwan:

> Traditional Chinese Medicine knowledge is often passed on by word of mouth... Soup made by boiling chicken with Traditional Chinese Medicine is delicious.

Traditional Chinese Medicine is often prepared with chicken, which makes the soup more palatable and less like a medicine. This man's early childhood experiences took place in a village where Western medicine was not easily accessible. Traditional Chinese Medicine was a family tradition: his parents used Traditional Chinese Medicine and his grandfather was a practitioner in Traditional Chinese Medicine. Whenever he had a health problem, his grandfather would come and look after him. His grandfather also planted herbs and used them both for medicine and for food. When this man grew up he continued to use Traditional Chinese Medicine and also planted herbs for food. This association between Traditional Chinese Medicine and food probably contributes to people feeling that Traditional Chinese Medicine is safe and free of side-effects.

This 58-year-old woman in Sydney (originally from Mainland China) had a fond attachment to Traditional Chinese Medicine, and continued the family tradition of using it as a food supplement:

> I have been using Traditional Chinese Medicine all my life... Traditional Chinese Medicine provided a means of looking after my children in my generation.

She had learnt how to use Traditional Chinese Medicine with her mother, who had been knowledgeable, and as a child she had continued the tradition by preparing Traditional Chinese Medicine for her younger brother and sister. Importantly, Traditional Chinese Medicine provided a convenient code for caring for her own children, mainly through various food preparations. She insisted on carrying on the family tradition, sharing her knowledge of Traditional Chinese Medicine on air as a part-time announcer on Chinese radio in Sydney.

Negative experiences of Traditional Chinese Medicine

The above sections present positive experiences of Traditional Chinese Medicine, positioned in a system of mutual obligation and connections. In contrast, people speak of negative experiences with Traditional Chinese Medicine in this section.

As a sign of 'rebellion'

A 48-year-old woman in Sydney (originally from Hong Kong) stated:

I had Traditional Chinese Medicine because of rebellion against power and control in the family.

Taking Traditional Chinese Medicine gave this woman the opportunity to express rebellion against the authority and injustices she experienced with her in-laws. Her dominating mother-in-law looked down on her because of her poor background. When she had first moved into the family, her mother-in-law had warned her: 'Don't you think you can do whatever you want to in my house'.

Her in-laws had restricted her freedom and attacked her, calling her a fool and using an old saying that denigrates women: 'Do not give enough rice to women before they turn eighty' (女人未到八十歲不要給她吃太飽). Moreover, they expressed contempt for her parents, saying that she had a 'dead father and dead mother, and no family education' (死老豆死老母親沒家教). This insult was enough to put her 'on fire', as she said, and her feelings turned to hatred and rejection.

During her pregnancy she was not given Traditional Chinese Medicine for nourishment. When she obtained it for herself, she was told: 'after taking this Traditional Chinese Medicine, your baby cannot come out'. Note this view that Traditional Chinese Medicine was so nutritious that it could increase the size of the baby. She persisted and took Traditional Chinese Medicine in the face of this opposition. Finally, when she gave birth to a baby girl, not valued by her in-laws, they did not give her Traditional Chinese Medicine during the 'resting month' (the period following childbirth when rest and good nutrition are traditionally recommended). She prepared Traditional Chinese Medicine for herself as much as she could to spite her in-laws.

Disobedience to parents-in-law is a sign of unfilial behaviour in traditional Chinese thinking. This woman took Traditional Chinese Medicine as an act of rebellion against their authority. In fact, this Traditional Chinese Medicine symbolised the parental love and reciprocal obligation that she was not getting!

Breaking with the social past

The following case, from a 76-year-old woman in Sydney (originally from See Yup, Mainland China), illustrates another negative experience of Traditional Chinese Medicine:

> I use chicken to boil soups and add Traditional Chinese Medicine. What I am afraid of is not death but the thought of becoming paralysed. I would not like to be taken care of.

She used Traditional Chinese Medicine in the belief that it could safeguard her health and preserve her independence. There are five aspects of her drive to remain independent: 'wrong birth', betrayal, unhappy family life, rebellion, and freedom.

Wrong birth. She considered that the time and place of her birth had affected her life:

> I was born in the wrong place... I was a cheap person with cheap bones (賤人賤骨頭).

A 'wrong place' is where all ill fate is generated. A 'cheap person with cheap bones' is a metaphor for an unworthy person with no social status.

Betrayal. She was betrayed by her sister and was later sold to a distant isolated poor village (where tigers could be found) as a child bride (a future bride looked after by the future parents-in-law until she grew up). People living in the village ate anything and everything to survive, including banana roots and papaya tree roots. She had rice only three days each year – Chinese New Year Eve, Chinese New Year, and the following day. For the rest of the year she had porridge (watery rice). She developed an aversion to porridge after eating it for such a long time:

I was sick of porridge after a few decades... I have tasted the sweet, sour, bitter, and nasty side of life... and I used to think, how can I have more rice to eat?

Unhappy family life. She gave birth to a baby boy but the baby died after six months. She nearly died giving birth because of insufficient medical attention. Moreover, she was frightened of the traditional Chinese healing which had caused her so much pain. Later, her husband died in middle age.

Rebellion. She rejected tradition, as illustrated by this rebellious 'unfilial' behaviour:

When my mother-in-law brought me Traditional Chinese Medicine, I threw it quickly under my bed. My mother-in-law wanted to hit me, and I fought back.

Her actions of disobedience, of rejecting Traditional Chinese Medicine and of fighting back, were unfilial and unacceptable in those days, yet she stood up for herself and succeeded in protecting herself from further harm.

Freedom (a break from her past). Her life resembled the classic Chinese stories – with sad beginnings but a good ending. She had left everything behind. She enjoyed her new life and freedom, saying: 'I want to be as free as a bird'.

If Traditional Chinese Medicine symbolises mutual and reciprocal obligations of filial piety, then rejecting Traditional Chinese Medicine clearly symbolises rejecting family and the social control that family obligations impose, and a bid for freedom.

Discontinuity of tradition

Some participants brought up using Traditional Chinese Medicine chose to discontinue its use later on.

Shift from animals to humans

As a child, a 35-year-old woman in Sydney (originally from Hong Kong) had a strong association with Traditional Chinese Medicine. Her father worked in a Traditional Chinese Medicine shop, and she learned Traditional Chinese Medicine from her parents who had also learned from their parents. Traditional Chinese Medicine was 'always there', whether they had money or not. However she ceased using Traditional Chinese Medicine because of the influence of her brothers, who were Western doctors, and because of her own experience as a nurse, leading her to feel she had moved away from traditional ways:

> Because of my work, I am not traditional. I seldom use Traditional Chinese Medicine now.

Also, she had shifted her focus from animals, which she had used to treat with Traditional Chinese Medicine, to people:

> I used to give Traditional Chinese Medicine to my pigeons. After I took up nursing I learned the value of human beings, and shifted to Western medicine.

She had kept pigeons at home and fed them with Traditional Chinese Medicine. Because of her interest in animals, she had first wanted to be a veterinary surgeon. Later she took up nursing where she learned the value of human beings who could communicate with her and express their gratitude and appreciation in ways that animals could not. The shift of interest and environment had led to a shift in her use of medicine from Traditional Chinese Medicine to Western medicine.

Out of contact with Traditional Chinese Medicine

In Hong Kong, the mother of a 45-year-old man in Sydney had frequently prepared herbal teas and soups for him, and he had given Traditional Chinese Medicine to his own daughter. It had been convenient to use Traditional Chinese Medicine in Hong Kong, where ready-made herbal drinks can be bought easily:

> I had Traditional Chinese Medicine herbal drinks because I heard other people saying that they were good.

However he had ceased to use Traditional Chinese Medicine after moving to Sydney. In Sydney he had found Western doctors to be more convenient, and he was unable to find the same ready-made drinks as in Hong Kong.

Reflections

This chapter has traced the social discourses of Traditional Chinese Medicine relating to family connectedness. The transcendent discourses of Traditional Chinese Medicine are created, shared and perpetuated through the symbolic integrity of family relationships. Traditional Chinese Medicine plays a symbolic role in human interactions where its use signifies reciprocal value – to care and to be cared for. Underpinning the giving and taking of Traditional Chinese Medicine there is the timeless devotion of maternal care towards children and of reciprocation in children's indebtedness towards their parents. Filial piety toward parents can be demonstrated by giving care or by material return, and both are valued. Filial piety is the core of Confucian values for creating social stability and harmony.

However, filial piety can also be depicted as a form of social control, best illustrated here by the cases where negative experiences with Traditional Chinese Medicine led to rebellion against the use of power in the traditional family system.

Another important role of the family is to pass on knowledge, both within a family and by interacting with friends. These acts of sharing Traditional Chinese Medicine extend the meaning of filial piety. Through Traditional Chinese Medicine, people are able to express themselves and to be socially acceptable. However, the two 'discontinuity' cases indicate the opposite – a break from the past.

The continuity of tradition, of which Traditional Chinese Medicine is a fundamental part, constitutes a social bond that holds family and generations together and gives meaning to life. In Traditional Chinese Medicine there is no clear line between food and medicine.

Family connectedness reaffirms one's social roles in the family and in society. Despite changing lives, family connectedness is socially and culturally constructed and context-specific, constructed in part by cultural practices such as Traditional Chinese Medicine. The following chapter deconstructs how various conceptions of social and cultural identities are constituted and practised through the discourses of Traditional Chinese Medicine.

chapter seven

Identity

(Pronounced as *tong*, which refers to identifying and sharing)

Identity and culture are inseparable, and identity is subjective and social.

Brah 1996

Introduction

The symbolic consumption of Traditional Chinese Medicine evokes the discourses of identity. Participants often used dualistic discourses, in particular to describe human relationships, which are socially constructed. Traditional Chinese Medicine was perceived as a form of 'cultural heritage' or 'Chinese treasure', embracing shared meanings of Chinese identity in the Chinese diaspora. The use of Traditional Chinese Medicine to enhance physical appearance designates a relationship with social identity. The metaphor of Traditional Chinese Medicine as 'strength' symbolises masculine identity. Binaries such as this are geared toward the archetype of Chinese dualisms, *yin* and *yang*, in terms of human relationships. Through identity, one is able to define the self, and to locate the self in relation to others. The human relational properties of identity and binaries are strategic concepts that are dynamic, changeable, and contextually and socio-culturally specific. For Foucault, this quest for self-understanding is a 'perpetual task' and 'the foundation of all human endeavour', and 'it is through creativity that our power is revealed, and it is in our capacity to use it well that our destiny lies' (Hutton 1988:139).

Concept of identity

Identity defines who we are, and it is socially produced through human interaction. Identity and culture are inseparable, and identity is subjective and social (Brah 1996). For Erikson (1968:19,20), identity refers to 'a subjective sense of an invigorating sameness and continuity… a unity of personal and cultural identity rooted in an ancient people's fate'. This identity is dynamic and subject to change through our various experiences in life. For Giddens and Foucault, identity is actively constructed and relational. Giddens (1991:52) refers to identity as the reflexive awareness and activities of the individual in connecting oneself and society. This process involves change, and is fluid and dynamic because of the impact of modernity. In *Technology of Self*, Foucault writes that identity can be found in self-knowledge (Foucault 1988); through creative practices such as writing, exercises and introspection, body and soul are linked (Rabinow 1994). Social interactions can include seeking spiritual guidance, during which a reciprocal obligation is formed as each party to this shared experience benefits. Foucault's proposition is that we can reshape our past and that we are not limited by it. The past serves only as a mirror and provides only a partial truth about our identities. The journey for self-understanding is a form of self-care and a creative process and, through affirmation in the present, the meanings and values of our lives are revealed (Hutton 1988:140).

Chinese identity

Chinese identity is associated with the term 'diaspora'. The Greek word diaspora, according to *the Penguin Atlas of Diasporas* (Chaliand & Rageau 1995:xiii) was used by Thucydides to refer to the exile of the population of Aegina. Later the term came to denote the forced exile of the Jews in Babylon (586 BCE) and then to the 'dispersion' of Christian communities across the Roman Empire.

In modern terms, diaspora signifies a dispersion of an originally homogenous people; in this book the term is used to refer to migrant Chinese people in Australia and the Chinese people in Hong Kong and Macau and their descendants. The concept of diaspora is embedded in the social, cultural, and historical dimensions of the immigrant experiences and settlers. Diaspora is associated with dynamic experiences of 'interconnections, nostalgia, memory and identity' (Wimmer & Schiller 2003).

In the Chinese diaspora, the sense of 'being Chinese' is argued to be a 'constructed identity' in which 'language, history, custom, beliefs and values occupy particular niches' (Chun 1996:54). According to Foucault, a homogeneous sense of national identity produces social solidarity; at the same time it restricts civil participation in cultural discourse and generates the possibility of different constructions of identity (Chun 1996:62).

Many participants in this study identified Traditional Chinese Medicine as being a fundamental aspect of being Chinese. They referred to its historical presence throughout Chinese history as well as its intimate role in their own life experiences.

Food as Chinese identity

The Chinese identity of the following two participants was experienced through Chinese food, involvement with the Chinese community, and the use of Chinese decorations in their homes. They were brought up in Australia and did not speak a Chinese language, so Traditional Chinese Medicine foods and artefacts had become their main links with Chinese identity.

In the experience of this 39-year-old woman in Armidale (originally from New Zealand), Traditional Chinese Medicine was associated with food:

Traditional Chinese Medicine means food to me. My Chinese identity is with food… I had my first Chinese meal when I was twenty-eight.

Her first significant exposure to her Chinese identity had come quite late. Born in Hong Kong, she had initially been looked after in an orphanage before being adopted into a Western family and brought up in Australia without a firm Chinese identity. In her presentation and speech, she appeared very much like a Westerner. In order to avoid becoming a social misfit, she had made great efforts to be socially acceptable: she dressed in a Western way, used foundation to have a complexion like a Westerner, and spoke English with a local accent.

Yet she was also seeking another identity as being Chinese: 'I want to know more about me. I want to know what makes me.' She decorated her home with Chinese artefacts (fortune stones and coins), cooked good Chinese food, and had a big wok. She even fed her rabbit with Chinese vegetables such as pak choy (白菜), which she believed made the rabbit look well.

Her quest for self-understanding and her reflectiveness are revealing. Bauman (1992:vii) suggests that identity is flexible and changeable in postmodern conditions, in which people have come to have the habit of reflecting on themselves, of searching the contents of their minds and reporting on what they find.

All things Chinese

Similarly, the participant in the next case was not brought up in the Chinese way. With a Chinese father who had little time at home, a Japanese mother and a Western wife, an Australian-born 69-year-old Chinese man knew very little about Chinese culture. Yet he had a strong affinity with Chinese things such as Traditional Chinese Medicine ointments and foods. When he was a child, he used to eat at his Chinese friends' houses. He learnt from his friends' parents about some of the healing properties of Traditional Chinese Medicine, including cooling the blood and herbal teas for fevers. In his home environment he had less experience with Traditional Chinese Medicine practices:

> Not much about medicine. Except if we had bruises or anything like that, we would rub on this cream made from Chinese herbal leaves and brandy, and nothing much else, mainly foods, herbs that we used, and soups made from Chinese foods.

It was through traditional Chinese Medicine remedies such as ointments and foods and through home decorations that he acquired his sense of Chinese identity:

> We now have all things Chinese, cutlery. We were only in contact with things my father would have used. My father was involved in a lot of things dealing with Chinese; people say that I do look like my father.

Significantly, through the influence of his father, who had been involved in many dealings with Chinese people in Brisbane, this man was also active in the Chinese community.

For these two Chinese people, Traditional Chinese Medicine was linked with Chinese food, which conjured up the image of being Chinese. Through food, Chinese identity was positively affirmed with fond memories of the past as well as a sense of belonging. Preparing and sharing food is a social practice and a symbolic expression of Chinese material culture, which provides shared meanings of living as well as habits that sustain identity (Edensor 2002). It has been said that 'continuous interaction with objects engages the senses and makes the body remember' (Edensor 2002:107). Furthermore, decorating their home environments with Chinese artefacts highlighted relational cultural elements. These human–object relations make their Chinese identification tangible for them – human and object became one.

Another point is revealed in these participants' search for identity. Their quests are active and reflective. The 39-year-old woman in Armidale was eager to learn about herself and about being Chinese. The 69-year-old man in Brisbane identified with his late father and his involvement with the Chinese community. For many Australian-born Chinese, their identity represents two worlds and two cultures (Shen 2001), and as Tu (1991:ix) suggests, 'learning to be Chinese is an attainment rather than a given, especially for minorities and the foreign-born'.

Searching for roots

Like the 39-year-old woman in Armidale, identity for the following 21-year-old man in Brisbane (originally from Hong Kong) entailed a change of ways and an active search within oneself:

> Being Chinese and Traditional Chinese Medicine are part of Chinese treasure. I should be proud of Traditional Chinese Medicine. I insist on learning some Chinese things. I shall learn Chinese calligraphy because I am Chinese… I have changed now and become more Chinese.

Traditional Chinese Medicine evoked a sense of being Chinese for this third-year university student, who had developed greater affinity for Chinese things while in Australia. All the Hong Kong Chinese people that he knew in Australia were Westernised. He began to search for symbols of his Chinese identity – a sense of his own culture. A sense of having roots arises out of life experiences and socialisation in childhood (Djao 2003). He thought it was important to learn about Chinese things for three reasons: firstly, authentic Chinese people should know Chinese culture; secondly, learning Chinese helped to refine one's character; thirdly, from a practical point of view, Westerners would not criticise him if he knew Chinese customs.

The process of searching for one's roots becomes a quest for identity (Lee 1991). His sense of alienation within the Westernised society of his Chinese compatriots led him to redefine himself. Cultural pursuits, such as Chinese calligraphy, are an expression of this reconstruction of self.

Unchanging thoughts on Traditional Chinese Medicine

The following two cases illustrate meaning and identity for Chinese people underwritten by Chinese history and heritage, such as Confucian thinking and culture. Here, Chinese identity derives from self-reflection and the will to carry on traditional Chinese ways. The salient features of a diaspora include memory that transmits historical facts and cultural heritage and, importantly, the will to transmit heritage in order to preserve identity (Chaliand & Rageau 1995).

The concept of Traditional Chinese Medicine as Chinese culture was deeply ingrained for a 45-year-old man in Armidale (originally from Beijing). Most of his education had been received in Mainland China and he knew Chinese culture:

> At the age of thirty, we set our direction; at forty, we are unaffected by environment. But my thoughts on Traditional Chinese Medicine have not been changed… Traditional Chinese Medicine reflects thousands of years of heritage of China.

In the first sentence he borrows from Confucius's *Analects* (Book 2, chapter 4). The original version was 'at thirty, I stood firm; at forty, I had no doubts'. Confucius was giving an account of his vision and direction at various stages in his life. This participant used these words to characterise his way of thinking at two stages in his life, but noted that his affinity with Traditional Chinese Medicine had remained unchanged. He took great pride in the cultural achievements of thousands of years of history, including the two famous Chinese Classics he mentioned: *Journey to the West* (西遊記) (Ming Dynasty 1368–1644 CE) and *Dream of the Red Chamber* (紅樓夢) (Qing Dynasty 1644–1911 CE). These two books recorded examples of Traditional Chinese Medicine. Significantly, he also drew a parallel between Traditional Chinese Medicine as culture and the Chinese classics.

My core being is very Chinese

Similarly, a 30-year-old woman from Brisbane (originally from Papua New Guinea) conceptualised her Chinese identity in traditional Chinese culture as represented by Confucius:

When I read Confucius in English I felt I was coming home. I understood everything straight away, and it was the same with Traditional Chinese Medicine. I do not feel and think Chinese in the sense that I do not think and speak in Chinese, but my core being is very Chinese, my spirit is very Chinese. I might learn about my Chinese heritage and how Traditional Chinese Medicine is involved in that.

In spite of her Western influence and outlook, her core spirit remained Chinese. She organised Chinese cultural activities in Brisbane, hoping to learn more about Chinese culture and her Chinese identity. She was prepared to look deeper into Traditional Chinese Medicine – 'Traditional Chinese Medicine is something that I have thought about for the past ten years' – because of its connection with Chinese heritage.

This sense of belonging is a common sentiment among Chinese people overseas, in the peripheral areas and in the frontier lands (Wu 1991:149). Two common sentiments can be identified: firstly, a sense of connectedness with the fate of China, and secondly, a sense of fulfilment in the cultural heritage handed down from their ancestors.

I do not see myself as Chinese

In a departure from these sentiments, a 32-year-old woman in Brisbane (originally from Papua New Guinea) felt a lack of common culture, which had been determined by her social environment:

The things I associate with Traditional Chinese Medicine are ointments and foods; otherwise, I use Western doctors in Australia. I am not in touch with Traditional Chinese Medicine; I do not feel any connections to Traditional Chinese Medicine. My friends say they do not see me as Chinese. I do not see myself as Chinese.

She did not associate Traditional Chinese Medicine with a sense of 'being Chinese'. Her sense of Chinese identity was lacking both physically ('not in touch with') and spiritually ('do not feel any connections'). She was comfortable in Western culture and accepted socially by her friends, which had a greater influence on her self-identity and sense of belonging than her Chinese genes.

Identity and body

Identity and body are socio-culturally constructed. The traditional Chinese view was that people's bodies were gifts from their parents, and therefore it was their duty to take good care of their bodies. Neglecting the body was a sign of being unfilial. The Chinese obligatory duty of caring for the body was advocated by Mencius as an element of filial piety:

> Of all that is held in trust by me which is the greatest? The preservation of my body.
>
> (*Li Lou,* part A, trans. Dobson 1963:138)

The Taoist view of the body was reflected not only in the metaphor, 'the human body is the image of a country' (Schipper 1993:100), but also in the body as constituting a social reality – the interdependence of a person, the environment and the nation – an important part of thinking in Traditional Chinese Medicine. Taoism also emphasised the inner world of a person over the external environment, that is, one was to refine one's character and take care of inner self first before taking action in the outside world.

In the postmodern view, bodies are not merely biological but are socially constructed and influenced by cultural discourses (Foucault cited in Gorden 1980; Bourdieu 1984), and the body can be an expression of one's identity. Bodies are also hotly contested social spaces, where complex signs of 'human fantasy and of human trespass' can be observed (Morris 1998:145). For Foucault, the body is associated with institutions and discourse, and power can be exercised through the body. The body for him also consists of the practices of the care of self. He maintained that the practices one uses alone or with others on their bodies or souls are 'to transform' themselves in order to attain 'happiness, purity, wisdom, perfection, or immortality' (Hutton 1988:18).

Goffman (1959) articulated another approach that focused on the body as socially constructed. Unlike Foucault, who was concerned with the investment of power and control of the body, Goffman was interested in bodily management as a component of social action. He wrote of the dual relationship between the individual body and society, that is, how self-identity was closely related to social identity. He argued that the individual body could be controlled and managed through the exercise of human agency in social interaction. Goffman also emphasised the ways in which people managed their bodies – the 'shared vocabularies of body idiom' (or non-verbal communication), referring to the presentation of the body such as through dressing, bearing, movements and position, or body language (Shilling 1993:82).

Bourdieu regarded the body as an unfinished entity subject to social, cultural, and economic processes. He proposed a theory of the body as a form of physical capital, attaching people's identities to social values regarding the size, shape, and appearance of bodies. This theory of physical capital is particularly applicable in his reference to the dominant social class, which considers the body as a project in social life. The belief is that the body is actively shaped and controlled by the development of skills and acts of labour, added to the investment of time and money (Shilling 1993).

Projected image and physical appearance are key components in the discourses of postmodern identity, with the belief that consumption increasingly focuses on the body as a vehicle of identity, a process in which 'desire is embedded and meanings are located' (Kellner 1992 quoted in Bocock 1993:102). For Foucault, the body was actively shaped and influenced by discourses, that is, interactions between people either as talk or text as social practices (Howson 2004:27).

The association of Traditional Chinese Medicine with the body emerged strongly from the interviews with participants.

Traditional Chinese Medicine for physical appearance

A 40-year-old woman in Armidale (originally from Hong Kong) used Traditional Chinese Medicine as a means of conforming to the social value placed on slimness:

> Bird's nest is for physical appearance. Some movie stars take it like an ordinary drink... Every time I go back to Hong Kong for a visit; I become very conscious of my weight. If you are in Hong Kong among all the slim people, you do not want to eat any more. Everyone is slim there, the slimmer the better. One has to look good, even if one dies.

Here, expensive Traditional Chinese Medicine is connected to the social status of movie stars. This woman was self-conscious about her weight, making comparisons with her past slim body in the context of normative social pressures: 'everyone is slim'. Although she had lived in Australia for a number of years, she returned to Hong Kong frequently and was strongly influenced by the 'slimmer is better' consciousness among her social relationships there. Certainly it appeared that slimness as being socially acceptable had overtaken the traditional view that 'fat is better' in Hong Kong. As in the Western world, the body becomes the target of control and discipline. Body images change and are shaped by social and cultural meanings conferred on the body (Howson 2004).

The appearance of her body had become a life-long project. Under the Western cultural influence in modern Hong Kong, she clung to the belief that it was important to look good, even until she died. This body image, she admitted, had been imbued in her mind since she was a child. It was further confirmed by social environments in which slimness was valorised, as in the Western world (Cash 1990). Foucault's view (quoted in Gorden 1980:57) is that the body is influenced by the social preference for 'slim' and 'good looking'. Goffman's (1968) analysis of stigma is that our bodies reflect the view and prejudices of society.

Traditional Chinese Medicine for appearance is again stressed in another account from a 56-year-old woman in Armidale (originally from Hong Kong), reflecting on social pressures in a society where looks are emphasised:

> Traditional Chinese Medicine helps to enhance physical appearance. Chinese people say that 'females pay attention to their appearance both for themselves and for those who care about them'.

This woman confirmed that some types of Traditional Chinese Medicine are used in the belief that they will enhance physical appearance. Women experience pressure to use their bodies as objects for others to appreciate, as pointed out by Shilling (1993). The emphasis on self-identity through physical appearance arises from social interaction, and serves as a mark of gender desirability. The body becomes a social relationship and interactions reflect a person's symbolic value in a society; this value constitutes and is constituted by society (Bourdieu cited in Shilling 1993).

Traditional Chinese Medicine and body control

The socio-cultural influence of the stigmatising body was articulated by the following two men in Sydney with their concerns about 'old age spots' and 'grey hair'. A 62-year-old practitioner of Traditional Chinese Medicine (originally from Mainland China) associated the Traditional Chinese Medicine movement regime of Qi Gong with good health and keeping young:

> Some people at my age have old-age spots, but I do not. This is because I practice Qi Gong. I mainly use Traditional Chinese Medicine such as exercise to keep my body fit. Good health depends on whether we have regular exercise, such as Qi Gong, marital arts, running, and swimming.

Training the body gives one a sense of identity and self control. As an element of Traditional Chinese Medicine, Qi Gong exercise is used primarily for preventive health care. Importantly, self-identity is expressed through Qi Gong exercise. Exercising our bodies is a form of discipline for maintaining self-identity in a modern society in the process of change, and preparing oneself to face that change. Giddens (1991:100) argues that our bodies can be reconstructed through technological advances and knowledge. In Bourdieu's view, the body is a physical capital through which one's identity can be invested and shaped (Shilling 1993). For Foucault (1986:71), the body implies relations with others and, in a given situation, each enactment of a bodily gesture reflects cultural ideas about appropriate conduct.

A 45-year-old man (originally from Hong Kong) had been heavily influenced by the Hong Kong cultural emphasis on appearance. He had resorted to Traditional Chinese Medicine in an attempt to maintain his identity in the face of change:

> I started to have white hair, which I found not very nice looking because I was still young. I brought a particular Traditional Chinese Medicine drink.

Shared disciplines of body image

The group views of the younger-aged group in Brisbane (originally from Hong Kong) supported and confirmed the validity of the individual data and provided an understanding of the contexts of identity and body image in various locations. The discussion revealed the use of Traditional Chinese Medicine for the body and links with identity, as follows.

Firstly, Traditional Chinese Medicine was seen to help to improve body image. They recognised that body appearance is perceived differently in differing social environments. The young Brisbane group suggested that body appearance in Australia was not as important as in Hong Kong. Even within Australia, people in Brisbane presented themselves more simply and casually than people in Sydney, who were more conscious of their bodies and 'dressed up like peacocks' when they went out.

Secondly, in Hong Kong the presentation of self was stressed in a business environment, in a blend of traditional and Western values. In Hong Kong, shopkeepers would address not only girls but also old women as 'pretty girls'. This form of address, in the form of 'handsome boys', could also be extended to males.

Thirdly, and significantly, the group linked looking bad to being socially unacceptable: 'If people look bad they may not be reliable, their background must have problems'. The implication was that one had to be responsible and conscious of one's appearance; otherwise, one would be judged and socially rejected. This linking of body and internal being is reflected in the Chinese saying that 'the body outside tells what is inside'. Similarly, in Western thought the material body is considered to reflect the moral character on the inside according to Foucault (1990). In *Care of Self*, Foucault suggests that body and soul are linked; the self is found in the 'principle of the soul' (1986:25). Body and soul are inseparable in the care of the self which constitutes a way of living throughout one's life.

The group revealed differences in gender and educational levels regarding body image: girls were more concerned with their appearance than boys, and participants studying at university were more interested in appearance than participants at high school.

Gender identity

In this study, some female participants identified themselves with masculine characteristics, for example, in relation to the social disadvantages of being female in a poor family, in the highly competitive business world, and under the influence of one's social environment. According to Connell (2002:65), gender meanings involve complex understandings, implications, overtones and allusions embedded in cultural history. Sarup (1996) argues that identity is socially constructed using symbolic language, including gender.

A recent analysis of attitudes toward women in Taiwan and China revealed that a significant percentage of women (41 per cent) would have preferred to be male, and only a small percentage (20 per cent) were satisfied with being female (Higgins, Zhang, Liu & Sun 2002 cited in Chia, Allred & Jerzak 1997). To understand this finding, we should consider Chinese cultural images of women–in–man and gender expectations which affect identity and social behaviour. As Plummer (1999:48) argues in a Western context, 'women get more leeway for not being conventionally feminine than men who don't fit conventional male roles'.

For Chinese people, the image of woman–in–man was socially acceptable and even valorised historically. In popular Chinese folklore, Shanbo Leung and Yingtai Zhu (梁山伯與祝英台), a male and a female, met during scholarly pursuits. Yingtai Zhu was disguised as a male, and her friend, Shanbo Leung, was unaware of her female identity while they lived and studied together. Another famous heroic story was that of Mulan (花木蘭) who took on the role of a male to join the army on behalf of her father, who had no son. These two cases attested to the advantages associated with manhood, which offered greater social mobility and freedom to fulfil certain social roles. Such themes recur in Chinese literature, music and film.

There was distinct differentiation between expectations of the sexes among the traditional Chinese. Under the patriarchal family system, females were defined to a large extent by their reproductive and child-rearing potential. Although this attitude has changed to some extent in modern times, the rigid gender differentiation, binding men and women in marriage and reproduction, remains (Coward 1983). Males are expected to be dominant and to head the family. Men have more control and choice, while women are expected to remain subordinate. This 'cultural devaluation of women' (Stacey 1983:45) subjects women to social control in the traditional Chinese societies. As in Western societies, this element of social control is closely related to power relations, which are inherent in all social relationships. Power relations consist of struggles and confrontations – positively expressed as transformation and support, and negatively as disjunction, contradiction and isolation (Foucault 1990:93).

Working like an ox

Consumption is a social activity, which differs between social groups (Bocock 1993). A 74-year-old woman in Sydney (originally from See Yup, Mainland China) linked the use of Traditional Chinese Medicine to low social status. She was brought up in a traditional Chinese society in which women, especially those who came from poor families, had subordinate status. She compared her experience of hardship to being like an ox:

> We did not have much to eat, not to mention deer antlers or ginseng. I did not even have a chance to see them. I used to work like an ox. I did not want to be a woman.

In her experience, her poor family background and low social status placed Traditional Chinese Medicine largely out of reach. 'Working like an ox' is a common Chinese expression for having a hard life. In her case, the simile of 'like an ox' brings to mind images of hard agricultural labour, working hard without complaint, and also of dehumanisation. In her family as well as in her social environment, males enjoyed greater privilege which was why she wanted to be male.

Like a man at war

Traditional Chinese Medicine was perceived by a 48-year-old woman in Sydney (originally from Hong Kong) as enhancing her energy, so that as a woman she could compete in the masculine world:

> Traditional Chinese Medicine helps to enhance my energy. I needed energy to deal with business, which is like 'fighting a war'. In Hong Kong the business world is 'darker than a ghost' (黑過鬼) and one is easily lost in that complicated world.

While working in Hong Kong, she used Traditional Chinese Medicine to gain strength, to have the energy of a man. The metaphor of 'war' for the business world conjures up images of danger, fighting, and cruelty. She experienced it as a dark and surreal world where one needed energy to maintain one's way.

Moreover, in her thinking the image of 'woman' correlated with 'weakness'. She made her eyebrows thick to look tough like a man:

> You should never consider me to be a woman. I have to make myself look like a man. I think I have 100 per cent male character.

She identified as male because she was trapped between two ideals: firstly, as 'a practical person', and secondly, as 'a traditional person'. To succeed in achieving her practical ideal, she believed she need to cultivate a 'business' rather than a 'pretty' look, to be tough and not like those women who aim to get 'a lifetime rice ticket' (長期米票), which means hunting for a man to depend on. Regarding her traditional ideals, she had been influenced by her mother who had taught her to be strong. When she was a child, her mother had told her not to depend on men. Her mother had scolded her father (targeting his weak character) by saying that he was not like a man, and 'worse than a woman'.

On the other hand, money was a powerful theme in her use of Traditional Chinese Medicine:

> I had Traditional Chinese Medicine because I had money. I thought that with money I could see the best doctors.

She had neglected her health and needed Traditional Chinese Medicine to boost her energy. All the time she was thinking of how to make money, and with money she thought she could buy health.

Her embodiment of gender was related to her personal belief, her family influence, and her participation in the business world dominated by men. All these power and social relations shaped her identity.

Having too little yin

A similar view, that Traditional Chinese Medicine provided strength, was shared by a 30-year-old woman in Brisbane (originally from Papua New Guinea). Moreover, she admitted that she had little *yin*, the female character:

> I use Traditional Chinese Medicine [as food] to adjust my energy and to keep me strong. I have little *yin*. I always wanted to be a boy. When I was little, there were more boys around. I just played with boys. I was not a sissy. I even cut the hair short on my dolls. I am too strong.

In Traditional Chinese Medicine terms, she saw herself as 'being strong', of having 'little *yin*'. When *yin* and *yang* are used in reference to gender, the idea of balance by combining the two sometimes transmutes into a fixed dichotomy. For example, Chinese people often refer to strong people as having *yang* characters and soft and weak people as having *yin* characters. In her case, she said it was a family trait: 'all my family… all my aunts are strong women'. Her two grandmothers were symbols of strength for her. One of them was like a 'dragon woman'. The other was also tough and had sacrificed her childhood in caring for her family.

Binary discourses

As participants' stories unfolded, they often ascribed *yin* and *yang* to binaries in human relationships. This section deconstructs the socio-cultural conditions that give rise to binary discourses in specific contexts.

Binaries are socio-culturally constructed (Thompson & Hirschman 1995). In Western thinking, although binary opposition suggests a mirror image relationship of equal opposites, it is often the case that one member in the binary has privileged status, such as in the binary divisions of good and bad, male and female (Greg 1996). When binary dichotomies such as gender are applied to human relationships, fixed or rigid stereotypes often result. People make assumptions based on these binaries, disregarding complex human behaviour and choice which are influenced by lived experience and social influence within a specific culture. As Hammer (1990) argues, the danger with classification lies in the 'potential to dehumanise' when we try to put people into certain simplistic categories. Understanding and open-mindedness help us to appreciate the complex world that underlies these binary concepts.

On reflection, binary thinking in the Western way is quite different from the original Chinese notion of *yin* and *yang* which, in *Tao Te Ching*, is not a dualistic approach. In *I Ching*, the cosmic force of *yin* was at first referred to 'the cloudy' and of *yang* as 'banners waving in the sun', as pictured as the bright and dark sides of a mountain or a river (Baynes 1965:lvi).

Yin and *yang* are not concerned with surface differences; they are not fixed and rigid categories but rather are dynamic and changeable. They form a continuum and are context-specific. Unlike Western notions of polarised binaries that are vulnerable to 'polluting' each other, *yin* and *yang* philosophy emphasises equality based on the ways of nature that neither has a permanent advantage over the other, that opposing forces can even foster and nourish each other as they co-exist, balancing and providing mutual support for each other. The Taoists' view suggests harmony, recognition of differences and co-existence, with all phenomena having equal standing and coming from the same source – nature.

From the participants' discourses on binaries, binary concepts are shaped by the social environment, traditional cultural ideas, balance in body and spirit, mutual understanding and considerations, and importantly, as complementary in co-existence in human relationships.

'False little boy'

The metaphor 'false little boy' as expressed by a 39-year-old man in Armidale (originally from Shanghai, Mainland China) uncovers socio-cultural assumptions relating to gender roles:

> Social influences may cause imbalance. Some females are brought up among their brothers and play with boys, and their behaviour may be more like boys too. This is referred to as 'false little boy' (假小子), according to a Chinese saying.

The metaphor 'false little boy' produces the image of a little boy who in fact is a girl. This metaphor was connected with this participant's social experiences in Shanghai, where he had heard the term in common usage. This reveals a view of gender roles as potentially fluid, subject to the influence of the social environment.

The Taoist precept in Traditional Chinese Medicine is that there is a close correspondence between human beings and the environment. The living environment can deplete *yin*. In such a case, the 'interconsuming' character of *yin* and *yang* was seen to be at work, in that when one aspect is consumed the other remains in relative excess (Hammer 1990). In other words, if *yin* is depleted, *yang* flows in to provide balance. Again, in the dynamics of *yin* and *yang* reality is relative, not constant, and is subject to change.

Sexuality and spirituality in yin and yang

Yin and *yang* bring together sexuality and spirituality, according to the 70-year-old woman in Sydney (originally from Singapore):

> *Yin* and *yang* emphasises sexuality. Sex is natural in life, but if you put sex as the first priority, then this is not real love. I think the spiritual aspect is very important.

This woman attached importance to the relationship being all encompassing. First she pointed out the importance of sexuality, which is without doubt an important component of *yin* and *yang*, given that it is an integral part of human life. According to *Nei Jing* (*Plain Questions*, chapter 2:15 and chapter 3:18): 'Human life is based on *yin* and *yang*', and 'The growth and development of all things on earth depend on the intercrossing of the energy of *yin* and *yang*.'

Sex could rightly be called a major sub-discipline of Traditional Chinese Medicine. One of the aims of sexuality is to contribute to the order and harmony of the body (Schipper 1993). This harmonious interaction is considered necessary for an open and positive attitude (Ruan 1991). It is suggested that the goal (to achieve harmony) is interpreted as the Tao of sex 'to calm the *qi*, to pacify the heart, to harmonise the mind' (Zhang & Rose 1999:177). This can be read as combining the spiritual and physical body in order to achieve balance. In fact, the major preoccupation in sexuality in traditional China regards reproduction; the related techniques and manuals address the right functioning of *yin* and *yang*.

However this woman mentioned sexuality in conjunction with spirituality. In Traditional Chinese Medicine, the body and the spirit are interrelated. *Nei Jing* (*Plain Questions*, chapter 14) states that body and spirit can be maintained if people follow *yin* and *yang* principles. Illness will result if one indulges in sex with endless anxiety, draining the spirit of energy.

There are Three Treasures of life in Traditional Chinese Medicine: jing, *qi*, and shen. Our concern here is with the first and the last. Jing is the male essence, the semen, that is said to be stored in the kidneys. Shen is the spirit. Together, they form the physical and spiritual levels. *Nei Jing* (*Plain Questions*, chapter 14:77) states: 'If one has shen, he is full of life'. The Taoist text *Classification of Therapies* speaks of the interrelationship between body and spirit: 'Essence transforms into energy, and energy transforms into spirit' (Reid 1996:9). The relationship between our physical and spiritual levels can be explained through the function of kidney *yin* with its spiritual dimension. We are said to have kidney *yin* and kidney *yang* in each of us. Kidney *yin* energy is responsible for the transmission of spiritual love and humanity, linking with other energies. People with balanced kidney *yin* are perceived to be realistic and rational, yet passionate regarding internal and external perfection, based on the love of people and common good (Hammer 1990:107).

Yin *and* yang *in family continuity*

Yin and *yang* relates to a binary concept as expressed by a 68-year-old woman in Sydney (originally from Shanghai, Mainland China):

> I think everything on earth needs *yin* and *yang* balance, otherwise something will go wrong. Man and woman get married and have children. Thus humans can be passed on from generation to generation.

Marriage, in her view, serves the purpose of continuing the family line and fulfilling filial obligations, reflecting traditional ideas. In *Mencius* (*Li Lou*, part A, trans. Lau 1970:127) is the dictum, 'There are three ways of being a bad son. The most serious is to have no heir'. Failing to produce a male heir is considered a major breach of conduct because the heir is responsible for continuing the family tradition in ancestor worship. Thus the past creates the future and the future creates the past!

The balance of *yin* and *yang* in the family produces *qi*, children, and is reflected in the traditional Chinese family ideal of 'four generations under one roof' (四代同堂). Blair (1993) suggests that the constantly changing nature of *yin* and *yang* reflects reality in traditional China. Because of this constant change, family stability and continuity are emphasised, with intimations toward immortality. Through family continuity, the spirit of one generation is believed to be passed onto the next generation.

A contrasting construction of *yin* and *yang* was given by a 50-year-old man in Armidale (originally from Taiwan):

Yin and *yang* in Traditional Chinese Medicine reflects the balance of male and female, which should be equal. Those people who talk of 'male dominance' must be discriminating against others. Male and female have different roles at home, which I call home management. Now society has changed. In Taiwan it is not uncommon for females to go out to work, while men stay at home.

The concern of the Taiwanese is based on 'equality' of males and females. In *yin* and *yang* theory, we are universal, and each of us has both male and female energies. They are complementary and form part of the whole. The Taoist way believes in nature and opposes 'male dominance'. *Tao Te Ching* (chapter 28) advises people to understand the strength of a male but to keep some of the qualities of a female, such as a receptive and caring attitude. This requires people to make a conscious effort to embrace difference, to undertake a creative process by combining the qualities of strength and humbleness in their interactions with the world around them.

We can also see the dynamic nature of change, which strongly reflects *yin* and *yang* principles. *Nei Jing* (*Plain Questions*, chapter 3) states that the exterior is *yang* and the interior is *yin*. In traditional Chinese societies people believed men should stay outside while women stayed at home. But according to this participant, 'society has changed' and now sometimes the outside/inside roles for men and woman are reversed. This is a dynamic response to a changing society.

Avoiding two captains at home

An 80-year-old man in Brisbane (originally from Hong Kong) had a different view and rejected the fluidity of *yin* and *yang*. He used a metaphor to convey the meaning of *yin* and *yang*:

I do not believe in *yin* and *yang*. My philosophy is if you marry, you cannot have two captains. At home if people do not like listening to each other there will be a relationship problem. So far, I am the captain.

Hawkes (1972) suggests that metaphor helps to stretch the language and to unfold new dimensions in our understanding of words. This was exemplified by this use of the 'two captains' construct, which conveys a sense of two strong characters in a situation where just one leader is required. Having two strong characters living together brings the risk of disagreement. This philosophy has a parallel in the Chinese saying, 'a mountain cannot harbour two tigers' (一山不能藏二虎), otherwise both will fight for leadership and power. The use of this metaphor suggested this participant didn't support gender equality at home. Although he had been living in Australia for sixty-six years and had married an Australian woman, his attitudes reflected Confucian thinking which favours male dominance. The *Analects* (chapter 17, verse 25) say, 'women and petty men are difficult to handle'. Social control was important in Confucian teaching; each member of a family had a specific role to play. A woman was not considered equal but was subject to three obediences: to her father when she was young, to her husband when she was married, and to her son when she was old. For a woman, listening is a way of preserving harmony in a family.

Comparing two generations

However, as in many cultures, the balance of power between men and women in Chinese families is not consistent across generations. The middle-aged group in Brisbane (originally from Taiwan) and the younger-aged group (originally from Hong Kong) had different conceptualisations of the *yin* and *yang* binary.

The middle-aged group took a broader view and showed a better understanding of *yin* and *yang* theory. They considered *yin* and *yang* as 'the wisdom of Chinese people'. They referred to *yin* and *yang* theory (the co-existence of *yin* and *yang*) by the saying, 'single *yang* will not survive, and lonely *yin* cannot grow'. However, the younger-aged group understood *yin* and *yang* more as a fixed principle referring to male and female relationships. They used the term 'rigid binaries' and blended Western binaries with Eastern *yin* and *yang* philosophy. According to the younger group, *yin* and *yang* meant heterosexuality, such that physical attraction for the opposite sex was considered natural.

The middle-aged group, however, referred to *yin* and *yang* as a balancing concept, such as its use in creating a 'holistic approach' in health: 'We cannot use one medicine to treat all parts of the body'. They took the same approach to variety in Traditional Chinese Medicine foodstuffs. In terms of human relationships, the Taiwanese group in Brisbane was aware of the importance of the right match of character types. For example, as characters, gold and fire do not match, but gold and water do match and 'lead to growth'. According to this group, in Taiwan it was common for people to use the name 'gold–water' (金水). Gold (sometimes simply referred to as 'metal') and water refers to categories of quality and relationship in the five phases in Traditional Chinese

Medicine: metal, water, wood, fire, and earth. Gold and water are considered mutually nourishing and promoting (Xu 2001), in the way that metal enhances the life-giving properties of water by permeating it with refined substances (Beinfield & Korngold 1991).

The differences in the views of these younger and middle-aged groups mirrored social and cultural differences in terms of their different backgrounds, ages, life experiences, and knowledge of *yin* and *yang*. The middle-aged group had attained university-level education and had many years of experience teaching in Taiwan. They knew about Chinese culture, and showed an interest in *yin* and *yang*. The younger-aged group, however, had little exposure to the philosophies underpinning *yin* and *yang*, and their reference to *yin* and *yang* was framed by their daily experiences and social interactions. Their conceptualisation of *yin* and *yang* was less organic than traditional Taoist teaching and was more akin to the rigid impermeable binaries prevalent in the West. Being younger and from Hong Kong, this was understandable. Their view was more of a hybrid between cultures, very much in accord with Hong Kong's history as a European colony.

Reflections

This chapter has explored the meanings people attribute to Traditional Chinese Medicine, particularly in relation to identity and binaries.

Traditional Chinese Medicine evokes collective Chinese identity in that it is inextricably linked with food, it is valued as Chinese heritage, and it is treasured as a cultural achievement. Traditional Chinese Medicine becomes a unifying force binding participants from diverse backgrounds.

Traditional Chinese Medicine also infiltrates and connects identity and body, a relationship that is subject to social and cultural influences. The symbolic meanings of Traditional Chinese Medicine – used for slimness, in the form of exercise to maintain the body, and for enhancing appearance – reflect social and cultural influences in relations with others (including seeing the body as an investment and for providing a sense of self-control in contemporary postmodern conditions). These are strategies for taking care of the self.

Females' identifying with males was seen as one strategy for living. In the participants' world, female identities are subordinated and devalued in the business world. Families of females are said to have more 'yang' qualities when their characters are strong like men. Males are perceived as to be 'strong' and 'powerful' and this carries over into Traditional Chinese Medicine philosophy and use.

The binary opposition of *yin* and *yang* as expressed in human relationships is considered on the grounds of qualitative differences arising from socio-cultural influences. In Traditional Chinese Medicine, *yin* and *yang* implies co-existence, complementarity, balance and dynamic change in relationships. *Yin* and *yang* emphasises 'naturalness' in sexuality, and highlights the spiritual dimension. Sexuality, the body, and spirit are interrelated as a whole.

Gender relationships are seen as complementary and flexible. However, at some points in Chinese history, such as in Confucius's time and in contemporary Hong Kong, in traditional Chinese families *yin* and *yang* defaults to a narrow binary concept of family continuity. The ideas of Tao and of Confucius are at odds with each other when it comes to gender roles.

The younger-aged and middle-aged groups expressed differing views on *yin* and *yang*, with the younger group expressing a concept of prescriptions about sexuality and gender differences, and the middle-aged group demonstrating a broader understanding of *yin* and *yang* as embracing complementary and balancing qualities.

In the next chapter, an example of the human dimension of Chinese culture will be represented by Traditional Chinese Medicine seen through the lens of various conceptions of leadership. This insight was gained through the voices of Chinese people in Macau and Hong Kong.

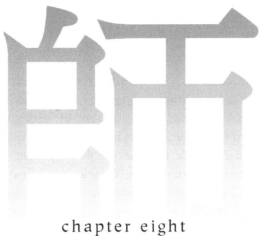

chapter eight

Conceptions of Leadership in Traditional Chinese Medicine

(Pronounced as *shi*, and means 'leader', 'teacher' or 'head')

Rod Gerber and Big Leung

The awareness of differences enriches us and makes us more human.

Big Leung

Introduction

Quality of health care, to a large extent, depends on good leadership. However, there is often a lack of leadership in health care (Bennis 2003). Understanding the dynamic human relationships associated with Traditional Chinese Medicine can help to improve quality of life, which was the impetus for undertaking the research reported in this chapter. For leaders in the health care environment, it is a challenging and meaningful experience to obtain knowledge of people's conceptualisations about the use of medicine, which are often influenced by health beliefs, personal experiences, knowledge and tradition, and are culturally and historically constructed (Leung & Gerber 2006). Understanding the various concepts, by sharing and listening to people, facilitates an effective service in the quality of health care delivery and outcomes. The aim of this research was to investigate the qualitatively different conceptions through which Chinese people in Macau and Hong Kong experience/think about leadership in Traditional Chinese Medicine. As an introduction, the concept of leadership in Chinese contexts is explored, including in the Chinese classics *I Ching* and *Tao Te Ching*.

Concepts of leadership in *I Ching* and Tao

Leadership is positively regarded in *I Ching* (易經), a metaphysical treatise about cosmic order and moral order. The principle of leadership is represented by various symbols. For example, the *Lin* hexagram ☷☱ (chapter 19) embodies some crucial elements of leadership: benevolence, righteousness, honesty, receptiveness, firmness and harmony. These elements are considered great blessings. At the same time, in practical terms good leadership should remain close to people, should choose the right people, and should use benevolence as a guideline for leadership (Chow 2005). The moral elements of sincerity and trust are highlighted in various chapters of *I Ching* (chapter 45, chapter 61). These elements set a guideline for good leadership in winning the hearts and support of people. Good leadership also radiates happiness, considered a great asset in attracting the commitment of followers. Moreover, leaders should be warned against insincere approaches from people and acting foolishly with them (chapter 58). Other winning attributes of leadership are humility and receptiveness. Equally important, however, is to combine these with firmness to maintain order (chapter 65).

Other examples abound on the Chinese concept of leadership. For example, in Tao teaching attributed to Lao Tzu (600–400 BCE) (chapter 17, Chung 2004), four types of leadership are classified from the point of view of the people:

- the preferred type of leader, less inclined to give orders and with a leadership style based on natural way (the Tao), such that people are hardly aware of the leader's existence
- a leader whom the people love and praise
- a leader whom the people fear
- the worst type of leader, whom the people despise.

The best leader acts in congruence with the Taoist teaching of self-discipline realised in non-intervention or *wuwei*. When a leader practises *wuwei*, the people may not be very conscious of the leader's presence. The concept of *wuwei* does not mean being passive, but rather it means doing things according to nature and harmonious relationships. It implies reflectiveness and awareness, and trusting people in allowing them more freedom and space.

This 'best' type of leadership did not exist in the ancient world of Lao Tzu, only in his idealistic world. However, the second type of leader did.

Qualities of leadership, according to Taoism, also include humility, which centres on the leader viewing the good of people as the prime objective (chapter 67). Another expression of humility is willingness to take a lesser role – the gentle and receptive role of a female, but with the inner strength of a male (chapter 28). The water symbol is used to denote flexible leadership (chapter 78); moreover, leaders should learn from the moral value of water, which is soft, willing to lower itself and to accept misfortune. The mastery of self embraces contentedness (chapter 33), advising leaders to 'know themselves but do not see themselves, take care of themselves but do not exalt themselves' (chapter 72).

Similarly, for Chuang Tzu (399–295 BCE), a Tao follower, leadership means to commit self to the Tao, as reflected in his paper 'Responsive Leadership'. Some dialogues on the Taoist way of leadership speak of displaying trust and acting appropriately (trans. Cleary 1998:116):

> If a leader personally expresses the norm and rules with justice, who would dare not obey and conform? Acting only when correct, making certain of the ability to do one's work.

The mental attitudes prescribed for leaders include being free and calm, simple and open, in harmony with nature, and unbiased. In other words, leaders should be unaffected by external forces and rely on inner strength, the way of Tao.

Study of Chinese conceptions of leadership

In the study reported in this chapter, focus groups of Chinese people living in Macau and Hong Kong were interviewed to explore their conceptions of leadership in Traditional Chinese Medicine. A phenomenographic research approach was considered appropriate for illuminating the underlying meanings associated with these people's conceptions.

People's conceptions are related to individuals and their surrounding world; the same phenomenon will be experienced differently by different people (Gerber 1996; Marton 1984 and Svensson 1997). According to Gerber (1992), phenomenography is a research method for mapping the qualitatively different ways in which people experience, perceive, understand or think about various phenomena in their world. This people-centred approach focuses on people's experiences, that is, the way people perceive and think about the world, regardless of the source of these perceptions (Marton 1981).

Results in phenomenographic research rest on the 'categories of descriptions' (similar conceptions shared by participants) and the 'outcome space' (the structural relationships amongst these categories).

Research questions

The interviews followed a semi-structured format using the following open-ended questions (with slight adjustment in Chinese translation) in order to shed light on participants' concepts and how they were related:

- What experiences have you had in leading Traditional Chinese Medicine practices?
- What have been good practices of leadership in Traditional Chinese Medicine?
- What have been the effects of this leadership on improving practices in Traditional Chinese Medicine?

Data analysis

The second author (Big Leung) conducted the interviews, transcribed the data verbatim in Chinese, and then translated the data into English.

We analysed the data using the phenomenographic aspects of the non-dualistic ontological perspective; the object of the research (qualitatively different conceptions of leadership in Traditional Chinese Medicine) and subject (participants' views of the object) are seen as related and not as separate. Regarding knowledge, we adopted the phenomenological epistemological position, which is intentionally constituted based on Husserl's ideas (as described in Sandberg 1997). The 'what' and 'how' aspects were used to explore the topic, 'What are the various conceptions of leadership in Traditional Chinese Medicine in these groups? And how are the conceptions related to each other?' Moreover, by 'bracketing' we set aside our preconceived positions and focused on the expressed experiences/conceptions, allowing statements to be constructed regarding what is understood as a result of these experiences (Gerber 2005).

Our interpretations of the data were made on a collective basis; we read the transcripts and defined each of the categories as a group, based on the context of identifying similarities and differences among transcripts and relationships between categories (Akerlind 2002). The aim was to capture the range of understandings within a group, not to capture individual understandings. Marton's (1986) account of phenomenographic analysis reads:

> The first phase of the analysis is a kind of selection procedure based on criteria of relevance. Utterances found to be of interest for the question being investigated... are selected and marked... The selected quotes make up the data pool which forms the basis for the next and crucial step in the analysis. The researcher's attention is now shifted from the individual subjects (i.e. from the interviews from which the quotes were abstracted) to the meaning embedded in the quotes themselves... A step-by-step differentiation is made within the pool of meanings. As a result of the interpretative work, utterances are brought together into categories on the basis of their similarities. Categories are differentiated from one another in terms of their differences... and finally are defined in terms of core meanings... Each category is illustrated by quotes from the data.
>
> (Marton 1986:42–3)

This research on Chinese people can only be understood within the contexts of Chinese studies, including Chinese philosophy, literature and histories, and so these contexts will be drawn on during the interpretation and analysis.

The participants

Each group interview took about three hours and was conducted in the participants' language of Cantonese. The twenty-four participants were divided equally into one group in Hong Kong and two groups in Macau. Fifteen were female and nine were male; fourteen were considered middle-aged (40–54 years) and ten were younger (17–39 years). Participants in the Hong Kong group, a mixed group of young males and middle-aged females, were students, teachers and a housewife, with educational levels ranging from high school to university qualifications. The educational levels in one Macau group, of mainly middle-aged females with one middle-aged male, ranged from high school to university graduates, with most of these participants working in commercial fields. In contrast, participants in the other Macau group, consisting of younger males with the exception of one middle-aged female, mostly had university-level qualifications and were working as social workers.

Conceptions of leadership in Traditional Chinese Medicine

Five categories of descriptions about conceptions of leadership emerged: as refining human relationships, as relating to self, as knowing the difference between the two medical models, as good management practice, and as embracing cultural environment. Within these, the groups focused also on a number of subcategories, revealing the complexities of these conceptions.

1. Leadership as refining human relationships

A consistent theme emerged that leadership in Traditional Chinese Medicine resides in human relationships. According to the groups, leadership 'is about human relationships' since the target is dealing with people This people-centred focus creates shared meanings by building trust and generating good emotions in human encounters.

Building trust

Confidence in human relationships is built on trust. Building trust can also serve in balancing power relationships. Trust between doctors and patients was discerned as paramount in Hong Kong where patients are powerless and have to listen to doctors.

> Leadership in Traditional Chinese Medicine is about dealing with people – the relationship must be built on trust, such as trust between doctors and patients. In Hong Kong, patients do not have much to say, they are like 'body on the chopping board' (肉隨砧板上), powerless, and have to listen to doctors.
>
> Hong Kong Group

Trust implies understanding and the right use of a leader's capabilities. Trust is shown by leaders delegating responsibility to followers. This gives followers the sense that they are considered important, and generates greater efforts from them:

Good leadership should trust and delegate responsibility and let followers make some decisions. It is important to allow some freedom, to empower people, so that followers can think and feel important and valued. In this way they would work harder.

Macau Group

Having high emotional maturity

'Emotional maturity' was highlighted as the main factor for good leadership. The view was expressed that people with good 'intellectual maturity' are generally poor in 'emotional maturity'. People with high 'intellectual maturity' may have psychological and social problems; they would tend to look down on people, resulting in 'social distance' between them and lesser educated people. The following quote shows the importance of 'emotional maturity' in generating reciprocal relationships:

Whatever the levels of leadership, the most important attribute is 'emotional maturity', not 'intellectual maturity'. If one can be on good terms with everyone to foster good human relationships, that certainly would impress everyone. As a result, people would help you.

Macau Group

On the other hand, good emotional display is seen as a natural gift for some good leaders who exhibit good *yuan* (緣). *Yuan* consists of two meanings according to the group: the luck in human encounter, and the way of handling people. A leader with good *yuan* would need to make no great effort to convince people, for people would naturally listen to such a leader:

If human relationships are excellent, there is no need for complicated handling. I think the most important attribute for leadership is *yuan* (緣). If your *yuan* is good, everyone would listen to you.

Hong Kong Group

2. Leadership as relating to self

Often the groups identified self as the foundation of good leadership in Traditional Chinese Medicine. Comments included 'leadership is all about an individual', 'if one does not know how to manage self, how then is one expected to manage others?'. Self was recognised as the building block of 'running a family, managing a country, and making peace in the world'

(齊家 治國 平天下). A good person embodying 'self' would exhibit exemplary personal attributes as well as having an attractive physical appearance.

Exemplary personal attributes

Personal qualities embracing good character, great efforts, commitment, and unfailing beliefs were essential attributes for good leadership in Traditional Chinese Medicine, according to the groups. Being open-minded was discerned as a most important aspect, and was cited repeatedly by the members of the three groups.

Also, leaders should not merely depend on rules from the past and take things for granted. In the following comment, this group suggested that leaders in Traditional Chinese Medicine should be open and aware of the complementary nature of Traditional Chinese Medicine in relation to Western medicine, and should understand that Traditional Chinese Medicine may not be effective for treating all illnesses:

> As a leader in Traditional Chinese Medicine, one should not merely think of Traditional Chinese Medicine as most powerful that can be applied to a hundred illnesses; a leader should be open-minded and realise that, to a certain extent, Western medicine is better.
>
> Macau Group

Similarly, a Macau group expressed the need for good leadership to be open and receptive to new and different ideas. In the experience of some members of this group, the practice of Traditional Chinese Medicine knowledge was too secretive:

> Good leadership must be open-minded and receptive to different ideas. In health service one must not only see the medical point of view, but open up your eyes in the surrounding environments, embracing the Eastern and Western mindsets.
>
> Macau Group

In the following account, the need for a leader to have personal acumen with sharp insight and awareness and an attitude of seeing things through was expressed:

> A leader in Traditional Chinese Medicine exercises personal style. This is not only about talent (天才), but also about one's capability of seeing

things through (通才). If one can understand one rule, one can understand a hundred of them (一理通百理明).

Macau Group

Having good appearance

An attractive image became a focus for the groups. Different themes are expressed in the two texts below: firstly, that appearance can be enhanced by dress, and secondly, that good clothes cannot disguise a bad heart:

> People in Hong Kong emphasise appearance. Being good looking is an advantage for leaders; people respect clothes first (先敬衣裳後敬人). A man must be dressed in a suit as a sign of leadership...

> On the other hand, one's face reflects the inside of a person. One cannot cover oneself entirely, no matter how well one dresses, like those with 'eyebrows and eyes of a thief' (賊眉賊眼).

Hong Kong Group

Another view was that good appearance alone is insufficient for good leadership, that leaders also need to have a good heart. The group gave as examples two prominent leaders in ancient China: Quin Shihuangdi (the first emperor in China) and Liu Bei (noted in ancient Chinese history as a wise leader with a good heart). The latter was remembered for his good and soft heart, apart from his strength, and the former for his cruelty:

> An attractive image is very important for a leader. However, just displaying physical attractiveness or being serious wouldn't turn one into a king, like Quin Shihuangdi, but one with the strength of iron and yet soft inside (鐵漢柔腸) will win, like Liu Bei.

Macau Group

3. Leadership as knowing the differences between the two medical models

The concept of leaders needing to know the differences between Traditional Chinese Medicine and Western medicine emerged, and of needing to consider the differences and the complementary roles of the two medical models. The groups focused on three dimensions of awareness: the differences between Traditional Chinese Medicine and Western medicine, the geographical environment, and the moral medical practice.

The terms 'fire inside me', 'high liver fire' and 'dirty blood' were used by the groups in the following two texts to describe bodily imbalances. Traditional Chinese Medicine was viewed as 'less strong' and also as distinguishable from Western medical practice.

Liver is reputed to support our emotional state and blood, according to Traditional Chinese Medicine. Any disturbance produces excess heat and causes bodily illness:

> Not too long ago, I wanted to scold people all the time. Once my pulse was felt, the Traditional Chinese Medicine practitioner said I had high liver fire (肝火上升), and asked whether I had been scolding people. I said I had.
>
> Macau Group

'Dirty blood' relates to the toxic material that accumulates in our bodies as a result of bodily imbalance:

> I used Traditional Chinese Medicine after feeling lethargic. A special needle was used on my skin. It was not acupuncture. The needle caused bleeding. Then a special equipment was used to absorb all my dirty blood. The theory behind that Traditional Chinese Medicine practice was to get rid of dirty blood inside your body, thus assisting body rejuvenation.
>
> Macau Group

In the following comment, the side effect of taking Western medicine was expressed in Traditional Chinese Medicine terms as 'dryness', arising from excessive *yang*. To balance this 'dryness', Traditional Chinese Medicine was used. The differences between the two medical models was seen to be in the rapid relief brought by Western medicine and in the time needed for therapeutic results in Traditional Chinese Medicine, as well as its balancing aspect:

> Taking Western medicine may cause dryness (燥). Western medicine is good for high temperature and Traditional Chinese Medicine as supplement.
>
> Hong Kong Group

> Traditional Chinese Medicine is not for quick relief. Rather it takes time for therapeutic purposes, and the meanings of balance or harmony are in Traditional Chinese Medicine.
>
> Macau Group

The need to appreciate the dualistic concepts of hot and cold in the geographical environment could be discerned. For example, living in a place where the water is hot may cause excessive heat in the body, so a herbal tea (a cold preparation) would be used to balance this. This group felt it is essential to understand the geographical situation when using Traditional Chinese Medicine:

> Place like Guangdong where water is hot, you have to take herbal tea to relieve heat. If you are in Hubei, Hunan, where water is cold, one has to take chilli to withstand cold. Good leadership needs to take into account geographical considerations such as water and land.

> Macau Group

4. Leadership as good management practice

The groups often equated good leadership with good management, because the target of each is people. Three attributes were considered important in good management: open-mindedness, sympathetic listening, and moral practice. The association between good management practice and good leadership is stressed in the following sub-conceptions.

Monitoring the right use of Traditional Chinese Medicine

The Hong Kong group expressed awareness of the need to monitor the effectiveness of Traditional Chinese Medicine. Considering the complicated nature of Traditional Chinese Medicine, many people may not understand the names of the herbs, the dosage rates, and how remedies are selected. As expressed below, good management should monitor the use of Traditional Chinese Medicine in order to safeguard human life:

> Good management is needed for Traditional Chinese Medicine, which is divided into heavy and light doses. Without sound management, medicine can be abused in use and may cause human death.

> Traditional Chinese Medicine formulas are complicated and patients should have the right to know what medicine is good for them, which one is for pyretic heat, and which one is for treating poisons.

> Hong Kong Group

Delegating responsibility

Good management was seen as making decisions and delegating responsibility. This does not necessarily mean knowing all the details, but it does mean supervising the overall plan of a large organisation.

> Good leadership needs to know management but one does not need to go into too many details, one can delegate others to take charge of works. It would be impossible for one to look after hundreds of people in an organisation.
>
> Macau Group

Moral medical practice

The focus on moral medical practice together with the need to make money was set against the background of the Hong Kong culture where, according to the group, 'people are more money conscious'. However, moral ethics were considered important in both Traditional Chinese Medicine and Western medicine practice, because people's lives are what is most important. Therefore, balance is needed to address the practical aspect of making money with the moral aspect of ethics:

> Traditional Chinese Medicine practice must make money too. [However], moral ethic in the practice of both Traditional Chinese Medicine and Western medicine is important. Balance is what we need.
>
> Hong Kong Group

Advancing health service

Good management was seen to improve the quality of a health service by facilitating health care in a systematic way, by using advanced equipment, and by getting capable people to share their experiences. With good management, health services are available and easily accessible, and patients do not have to go far:

> Good management can handle things systematically, and can convince the public... This is management – there is advanced modern medical equipment in Macau, and specialists can be employed from Hong Kong for operations if needed. Patients do not have to go to Hong Kong.
>
> Macau Group

5. *Leadership as embracing cultural environment*

All three groups strongly emphasised the need to understand the cultural environment within which a practice of Traditional Chinese Medicine is embedded as being fundamental to good leadership in this field.

The influence of being former Western colonies was seen to have resulted in a higher preference for Western medicine in Macau and Hong Kong. People know more about Western practices because of their exposure to them:

> Leadership in Traditional Chinese Medicine is about history and culture... Traditional Chinese Medicine is deeply rooted in Chinese societies. Because of the geographic influence of Macau and Hong Kong, which are more under the influence of Western practice, most people use Western medicine.
>
> Macau Group

In the same group, Macau's proximity to Mainland China was seen to increase sales in comparison with Hong Kong:

> People in Macau use Traditional Chinese Medicine more than the people in Hong Kong. The relationship of people in Macau with Mainland China is closer, which is reflected in sales.
>
> Macau Group

Traditional Chinese Medicine was understood as Chinese culture, so leaders in Traditional Chinese Medicine should have a deep understanding of Chinese culture. The group also took a global view that Chinese culture can be transmitted to the world through Traditional Chinese Medicine:

> Good leadership in Traditional Chinese Medicine should know Chinese culture ... Through Traditional Chinese Medicine, Chinese culture can be transmitted to the world, because Traditional Chinese Medicine is Chinese culture.
>
> Hong Kong Group

In another comment by this same group, leaders in Traditional Chinese Medicine are called on to recognise the fast pace of life in Hong Kong, and to respond by producing quick results:

> Good leadership should know that the environment in Hong Kong is fast, and time-saving devices are important. Good Traditional Chinese

Medicine must be fast in order to adapt to the fast pace of Hong Kong society, where people expect Traditional Chinese Medicine to produce quick results.

Hong Kong Group

Elements connecting conceptions of leadership

Through the process of seeking the relationships among the various conceptions, taking into account the content, contexts and cultural meanings, four connectors were captured in the outcome space: the people-centred element, the moral element, the affective element, and the scientific thinking element. Significantly, underlying these connectors we can uncover some profound core values of Chinese culture. Results will be presented as discussion and in a table, a feature of the phenomenographic approach.

A. People-centred element

A common thread running through the texts of the three focus groups is the 'people-centred' element. For the groups, nothing was more important than people as far as leadership in Traditional Chinese Medicine is concerned, as exemplified by prioritising 'people' in Conception 1 (leadership as refining human relationships). Building trust and delegating responsibility are the two main concrete acts that bind people together. This is linked with Conception 2 (leadership as relating to self) in that 'self' is the foundation of Conception 1 in all relationships between people. Similarly, having good appearances in leadership is relational – appearances are for others to appreciate. In Conception 3 (leadership as knowing the differences between the two medical models), the harmony that underlies the appropriate use and application of each of the medical models is also people-focused, in that people's problems and needs must be appropriately recognised and responded to. The patient-centred ideal of good management practice in monitoring the effectiveness of Traditional Chinese Medicine is notable in Conception 4 (leadership as good management practice), with the aims of safeguarding human life and providing patients with better information; again, the lives of people are considered most important in moral medical practice. Finally, people become the focus of cultural and environmental concern in the use of medicine in Conception 5 (leadership as embracing cultural environment).

B. Moral element

Good leadership in Traditional Chinese Medicine was often depicted by the groups as being embodied by an 'all rounded person', a person with a holistic perspective, and the moral dimension was given high preference. Conception 2 (leadership as relating to self) is replete with the moral element of good leadership with the leader as a 'good person': having exemplary personal attributes, cultivating self, having awareness, and possessing a good heart. A 'good self' is a requisite for 'running a family, managing a country, and making peace in the world' (from *The Great Learning*), as quoted by one group. This moral self is linked with Conception 1 (leadership as refining human relationships) by the use of 'trust' as a basis for human encounters. This is also linked with the medical practice in Conception 4 (leadership as good management practice) implying the importance of ethical practice in Traditional Chinese Medicine and in Western medicine, and with the moral responsibility for human life and the need to monitor the effectiveness of Traditional Chinese Medicine.

C. Affective element

The affective element can be indirectly related to A. (People-centred element) and B. (Moral element) above. This is most prominent in Conception 1 (leadership as refining human relationships) with the view of good leaders as having high 'emotional maturity' which helps in 'fostering good human relationships', and *yuan* (緣), the intuitive feeling or luck that binds people together. In addition, followers 'feel' empowered and 'valued' when good leaders delegate some freedom and responsibility. One group linked this affective element with Conception 2 (leadership as relating to self) by drawing a parallel between one's face (external appearance) and one's inside feelings. Another affective view in Conception 2 was the use of 'the strength of iron outside and softness inside' metaphor, evoking the image of a good leader as not merely possessing a strong physical body on the outside (as iron) but also a soft heart inside.

D. Scientific thinking element

Traditional Chinese Medicine was sometimes perceived by the groups as being too reserved, not scientific enough, and too secretive. The attributes of open-mindedness and receptiveness were therefore considered imperative for breaking this barrier, as suggested in Conception 2 (leadership as relating to self).

This would require a radical change in thinking and practice in Traditional Chinese Medicine, namely, to embrace Western medicine and, to some extent, Western scientific practice, as indicated in Conception 3 (leadership as knowing the differences). This is also apparent in Conception 4 (leadership as good management practice) when introducing scientific management practices implies using advanced modern technology, and in Conception 5 (leadership as embracing cultural environment) when open-mindedness will be required to transmit Traditional Chinese Medicine knowledge to the world,

The relationships between the five conceptions are listed in the table at the end of the chapter on page 170.

Discussion and reflections

The three connectors of people-centredness, morality and affection are identified as some of the core values of traditional Chinese culture (Lam 1995; Leung 1989; Yu 1994). The definition of 'culture', according to *I Ching*, centres on people (Qian 1979:99, and see also chapter two above about the meaning of Chinese culture). The emphasis on people was echoed in *Mencius* (c. 371–289 BCE): 'the people are the most important, the country is less important, and the emperor is least important' (*Tsin Sin,* part 2, chapter 14) (民為貴, 國家為次, 皇帝為輕). Chinese culture is based on humans and their relationships, and the starting point is the individual. This is maintained in *The Great Learning* (chapter 1, section 5), a Chinese Classic handed down by the Confucian School, where the cultivation of self is prescribed in order to achieve 'running a family, managing a country, and making peace in this world', as quoted by a group in this study. An expansion of self becomes the motivating force for realising *yen*, which is 'humaneness' or 'benevolence', the highest ideal in Confucian teachings (Yu 1994). The pursuit of an ideal character (and also of an ideal world) highlights the values of humans, and the meaning of life depends on humans trying to act their very best in this present world. The focus of Chinese leaders, historically, was therefore centred on people and how a harmonious society could be achieved (Lam 1995).

Inseparable from this people-centredness is morality, which serves to provide a harmonising effect and gives new strength to this world (Yan 1988). The emphasis on morality (or virtue) is reflected in the teachings of Confucianism, Taoism and Buddhism. Again, *The Great Learning* (chapter 1, section 1) emphasises the importance of acquiring the knowledge of virtue (morality) as a requisite for the ancient learner, 'what *The Great Learning* teaches, is… to illustrate illustrious virtue…' (大學之道在明明德). The cultivation of self is based on morality (Lam 1995; Yu 1994), as well as being the main consideration of leaders who have the good of people as their prime objective (Lam 1995). In Taoist teaching, leadership is constituted by the *yang* (strong) or masculine aspect of leadership as well the *yin* (soft) or feminine aspect of leadership (Heider 1985). *Yen* or humaneness, the highest morality, is exemplified in 'trust' (as suggested by a group in this study), a foundation for human relationships and society (Yan 1988). Trust is the embodiment of a perfect virtue, securing compromise between humans, and one of the main attributes of enduring human relationships (Wong 1995). The nature of Chinese culture tends to be subjective and inwardly directed, emphasising morality and the cultivation of self, instead of being objective and scientific (Qian 1993). This is evident in the writings of the ancient Chinese philosophers and historians which are replete with moral teachings like 'humaneness', 'righteousness' and 'loyalty' (Lin 1977).

Closely related to people-centredness and morality is the affective element, the 'roots' of Chinese culture (Lam 1995). Considering that traditional Chinese culture put human lives at the centre of attention, it is understandable that the moral element of *yen* or humaneness is imbued with the affective element. For example, Mencius believed that human nature is essentially good and full of feelings, as illustrated by his example of seeing a child about to fall into a well, mentioned in the previous chapter.

In reading Chinese classical philosophy or literature, in fact, the finest Chinese classical literature, we find that rich meanings of affection and deep human feelings abound, not merely between humans and humans, but also between humans and their environment; everything on this earth can be assigned to affective thinking and concern. Without this affection, *yen* would be meaningless and artificial. Traditional Chinese culture is regarded as an 'affective culture' (Lam 1995) as reflected by the principles of respect for the elderly and care for the young, filial piety between parents and children, and loyalty to work and superiors. These guiding principles give people strength. As Qian (1979:110) has expressed: 'as long as we have loyalty and filial piety, though home once destroyed can be rebuilt again; though a country was perished can be survived once more'.

Overall, conceptions of leadership in Traditional Chinese Medicine unfold some of the manifold and dynamic human relationships embedded in social,

TABLE: Relationships Between the Five Concepts of Leadership in Traditional Chinese Medicine

Core variations	Connectors	1: As refining human relationships	2: As relating to self	3: As knowing the difference between the two models	4: As good management practice	5: As embracing cultural environment
CHINESE CULTURE	People-centred element	Dealing with people, trusting and delegating responsibility	Self, the foundation of all human relationships, good appearance, linking with others	Understanding harmony in Traditional Chinese Medicine	Monitoring the effectiveness of Traditional Chinese Medicine to safeguard people	Medicine being used by people in various cultural environments
	Moral element	Trust, relationships and responsibility cultivating self, having awareness and a good heart	Moral responsibility for human life			
	Affective element	Having emotional maturity, good yuan, followers 'feeling' valued	A person's face reflecting the inside feelings			
WESTERN MODERN CULTURE	Scientific thinking element		Being open-minded, receptive to Western medicine, ideas and practice	Understanding the differences between the two medical models	Using advanced modern technology in management practice	Transmitting Traditional Chinese Medicine knowledge to the world

cultural and historical contexts. Understanding obtained from these views helps us to appreciate the leadership of Traditional Chinese Medicine in health care and in our lives as a whole. It is the awareness of differences that enriches us and makes us more human.

Throughout this book, the theme has emerged that Traditional Chinese Medicine is a social and cultural system, clustered around at least the six significant discourses developed in chapters two to seven. Each of these defining discourses highlights aspects of the human dimension in Traditional Chinese Medicine, as well as shared and overlapping meanings.

The focus of the final chapter is to draw the connections among the six discourses by means of their social and cultural significance.

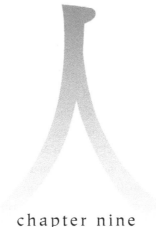

chapter nine

The Human Dimension

(Pronounced as *yen*, refers to benevolence and human dimension)

There are two things in China that have made significant contributions to this world: Traditional Chinese Medicine and Chinese food.

Mao Zedong (as quoted in *Mingpao* newspaper 2003)

Introduction

The social and cultural meanings of Traditional Chinese Medicine as drawn from participants' contributions uncover the human dimension of Traditional Chinese culture: the love of life focusing on this present world, the care of self in preserving health, the commitment to filial piety by showing reverence to parents and seniors, caring for the young, admitting co-existence while permitting differences in the harmonious and complementary relationships, trust and respect in social relations, and through the non-dualistic belief of equality in Yin and Yang philosophy that permeate our lives. These humanistic core values have upheld the integrity of Chinese culture and cement social interactions, and their application can have a positive impact in this modern world.

In the hearts of the participants, the material object of Traditional Chinese Medicine as food has been transformed into human expressions and connections. As food, Traditional Chinese Medicine assists with realising the inner self as well as acting as 'social cement' in a way that facilitates interactions at all levels of social life, in the family and in wider society. Significantly, Traditional Chinese Medicine embodies the human dimension in relation to self and with others, helping to establish identity, maintain balance, and unite all into a whole. These core values of traditional Chinese culture underlying Traditional Chinese Medicine are explored in this final chapter.

Traditional Chinese Medicine as food

Participants often talked about, understood, and related to Traditional Chinese Medicine as food. Indeed, according to many participants, Traditional Chinese Medicine meant 'food', and as such was connected with social and cultural identities as an expression of social cohesion and in the integration of social groups. The metaphor 'Traditional Chinese Medicine as food' emerged repeatedly throughout the analysis.

Chinese people have a long history of using foods for prevention and health promotion. A popular Chinese saying is that 'illness comes from the mouth'. As far back as the Qin Dynasty (221–207 BCE), food was related to as medicine and was considered superior to specific medical treatments. People believed 'food therapy is better than medicine therapy'. Sun Si-miao (581–682 CE), the famous Chinese physician from the Tang Dynasty (618–907 CE), commented on the importance of using foods before medicine for managing disease:

> A true doctor first finds out the cause of the disease, and having found out, he tries to cure it first by food. When food fails, then he prescribes medicine.

> (Lin 1938:255)

Food as medicine is consumed both in order to prevent disease and to ensure health. The boundary between Traditional Chinese Medicine and 'food' is unclear, and indeed food and Traditional Chinese Medicine together constitute a continuum. The continuity between Traditional Chinese Medicine and food is understandable, given that both are considered important parts of Chinese culture with a common origin. Mao Zedong, previously

Chairperson of Communist China, once remarked that there were two things in China that had made significant contributions to this world: Traditional Chinese Medicine and Chinese food (*Mingpao* 2003).

An essential concept of Traditional Chinese Medicine is the close correspondence between food and energy (or *qi*). Traditional Chinese Medicine was conceptualised by many Chinese people as the vehicle through which energy (or *qi*) in our bodies can be replenished, for strengthening *yang* energy for active boys, for male virility, for realising the social role of reproduction as in the use of Traditional Chinese Medicine soup for 'child bearing', and for health preservation and longevity.

Significantly, Traditional Chinese Medicine as food provides a crucial form of 'social cement' through which human cohesion, affection and social support are expressed, most often in social action. This is congruent with the views of traditional Chinese philosophy and Confucian teachings, which emphasised action; all reasonable knowledge of human behaviour, if not expressed through action, was considered mere empty talk. Fundamental to the social interactions is realising the value of self in Traditional Chinese Medicine.

'Social cement' in social interaction

Traditional Chinese Medicine as 'social cement' is realised in action, using Traditional Chinese Medicine as food to cement the three stages of human life (youth, adulthood and old age), as well as social relationships in the categories of parents and children, friends, gender roles and identities. Traditional Chinese Medicine as food also facilitates social interaction by means of social practices which act to establish conformity to social roles and norms within a family or in society.

In the family

Family is the first and most important place for realising social roles. Traditional Chinese Medicine as 'social cement' is most noticeable in the accounts of mother–child bonding through the mothers' preparation of Traditional Chinese Medicine to support their children. Children showed filial piety by remembering and practising the Traditional Chinese Medicine wisdom passed on to them by their parents, offering Traditional Chinese Medicine to their parents to show their care. Traditional Chinese Medicine as food is used within the family to maximise vigour and vitality in youth, adulthood and old age, and for preventive health care and a productive long life.

Traditional Chinese Medicine as a tradition is shared by families from diverse backgrounds. Traditional Chinese Medicine prepared as soup and shared among family members re-unites participants who may have moved far from their early lives in Mainland China, Taiwan, Hong Kong, and Papua New Guinea.

Friendship is expressed through the giving and sharing of Traditional Chinese Medicine, and in the giving of prepared foods to a new mother during her resting month.

All these interactions provide social cohesion by ensuring the continuity of traditions through the family and of the family through reproduction. Conformity to social norms and beliefs is reflected in the relations of Traditional Chinese Medicine to the social practices of sexuality and spirituality in the participants' social world. On the one hand, sexuality is narrowly defined as upholding the reproductive function of continuing the family line; other forms of sexuality are marginalised. On the other hand, the emotional and spiritual dimensions are also present, in that they permeate the concept of holistic balance.

In society

Traditional Chinese Medicine cements social identities and cultural identities. Social identity is established through gender roles, which are constructed and displayed through social interaction. Again conformity is discernable in a society where male strength is highly valued. Gender roles are deployed through the Traditional Chinese Medicine philosophy of energy. It is revealing that females who identify with male characteristics commonly used Traditional Chinese Medicine as food to enhance their masculine energy, to make themselves strong and effective in the masculine (business) world. Underpinning this social practice is the belief that women are weak; if one wants to be successful, one has to be 'tough like a man'.

The use of Traditional Chinese Medicine as a strategy for conforming to social norms is illustrated by attempts to enhance physical appearance, such by avoiding greying hair. Traditional Chinese Medicine is used for social acceptability in a society which emphasises appearance. This emphasis on appearance is culturally constructed and relational. Traditional Chinese Medicine as a social pursuit creates a bridge to others in the sense of it being 'for themselves and for those who care about them'. This is seen further in the belief of 'the slimmer the better', where the shift in acceptability from being fat to being thin has been facilitated by Traditional Chinese Medicine praxis. On the other hand, insufficient energy would mean a restricted social life and isolation, parallel with 'imprisonment'.

For cementing cultural identities, Traditional Chinese Medicine as food is considered as Chinese culture. Traditional Chinese Medicine evokes Chinese identity because it is a Chinese cultural 'treasure'. Findings reveal participants' reconstruction of identity and their search for 'authentic' Chinese culture and an authentic sense of Chinese cultural identity through Traditional Chinese Medicine praxis, which provides them with material evidence of that culture and identity have been internalised. Through tangible contact with Traditional Chinese Medicine as food, the intangible Chinese identity is positively affirmed, binding together Chinese people from different places of origin through shared cultural bonds.

As social facilitation

Traditional Chinese Medicine 'lubricates' social interaction by bringing people together. The element of exchange in social interactions is apparent. The role of exchange in cementing parent–children relationships is revealed when a mother prepares and presents Traditional Chinese Medicine soup to her children 'with her heart in it', and when children show tangible respect and gratitude, sometimes in the material form of money.

Traditional Chinese Medicine also lubricates social interactions with friends. Reciprocal social action is noted in the example of a participant who learned Traditional Chinese Medicine from parents and teachers in China and who, after migrating to Australia, continued to plant Traditional Chinese Medicine plants to share with friends as food.

Reciprocal social action contributes to social harmony and sustainability. The participants believed in filial piety, mutual support, caring for and being cared for in return, as illustrated by these comments by a 50-year-old woman in Sydney (originally from Hong Kong):

> My mother used Traditional Chinese Medicine for soup. She would prepare me pork heart with Traditional Chinese Medicine when I had an examination. The purpose was to calm my examination fears. I have a strong adherence to family tradition; I give money to my mother when I get paid and buy things for her.

Embodying the human dimension

Traditional Chinese Medicine: The Human Dimension reveals rich and profound values in Chinese culture manifested at all levels of life, including the reciprocal care of filial piety, trust, respect, considerations for others, the quest for self-understanding, and striving for peace and harmony. These inner virtues in human relationships offers a soothing refuge from and solution for the modern world which is often punctuated by imbalance, overdependence on material acquisition, distrust, violence, and man's inhumanity towards man. An understanding of the complexities of Traditional Chinese Medicine in terms of social, cultural and historical meanings enhances our awareness and appreciation of Chinese culture, which rests on deep human affections.

The human side of Traditional Chinese Medicine reveals profound Chinese cultural values in diverse social phenomena and cultural contexts. They are exemplified in four areas of social actions:

- cultivation of self, with various attributes associated with self-improvement, appearance, concepts of self in leadership, and self care,
- relationships with others, including within the family, between doctors and patients, and in the transmission of knowledge about Traditional Chinese Medicine,
- identities relating to culture, being Chinese, and consumption of foods, and
- balance, including the concepts of *yin* and *yang*, co-existence, and unity of the parts and the whole.

Together, they transform the material dimension of Traditional Chinese Medicine into something human and enduring, and create a social understanding of Traditional Chinese Medicine as culture.

Cultivation of self

Participants' practices of Traditional Chinese Medicine reveal the utmost strength being applied in continuously striving for self-improvement and thus life. Traditional Chinese Medicine was seen a means for improving body image and appearance, as suggested by younger-aged participants and also, in particular, by female middle-aged participants, whose perspective was that the outside reflects the inner self. Younger-aged participants also used Traditional Chinese Medicine for the purpose of enhancing learning for a better self and future social roles.

Traditional Chinese Medicine in the form of exercise was used by middle-aged participants to search for the meaning of one's life, for self-discipline, and for achieving peace inside and harmonious relationships with the world outside. These participants also perceived self-care through the use of Traditional Chinese Medicine as being for the purpose of promoting future reproduction and virility.

Traditional Chinese Medicine was used for the preservation of self in terms of their health by the elderly participants. They listed their health regimes for taking care of themselves, which included taking Traditional Chinese Medicine soup, practising harmony in life, adhering to nature, leading a simple and humble lifestyle, and maintaining a positive mental attitude. All these practices reflect participants' self-reliance, independence and consideration for others (not to be a burden), and thus their love of life.

In short, self care and preservation of health is a creative and positive expression of intellectual maturity and love of life.

Important insights are also drawn from participants' attributes of self associated with leadership in Traditional Chinese Medicine. They embrace a holistic view of mind and body, including emotional maturity (which minimises social distance), open-mindedness, awareness, having *yuan* (luck in human encounters), and good appearances. Traditional Chinese Medicine is also used for enhancing one's personal appearance (appearance is relational – for self and for others to appreciate).

Relationships with others

Relationships with others are grounded in social harmony with the aims of achieving balance and living a positive, receptive, honest and happy life. The role of Traditional Chinese Medicine underpins the continuity of the Chinese family line. Maintaining the traditions of Traditional Chinese Medicine is seen as a means of securing permanence despite change and of honouring the past. Reciprocal filial piety, a key part in Chinese culture, is enacted through Traditional Chinese Medicine used as a vehicle for realising care, support and reverence in social relationships. Chinese family systems are people-centred, resting on affection and emphasising present life, action, and harmonious social relationships. Life and medicine are intertwined. The symbolic expression of family life through Traditional Chinese Medicine challenges us to think what it means to be human in a mutually respectful way and how to live in caring social relationships.

Outside the family, it has been demonstrated that the role of leadership in Traditional Chinese Medicine should be built on trust, such as between doctors and patients. Trust assists in balancing this inherently powerful relationship, contributing freedom and empowerment.

Another social interaction is the transmission of knowledge about Traditional Chinese Medicine, which again depends on a trust relationship between teachers and students as well as the unselfishness and openness of teachers, filial piety, awareness of Traditional Chinese Medicine, and students' willingness to work hard.

Identities

In the area of identity, Traditional Chinese Medicine is conceptualised as a 'cultural treasure' which is deeply grounded in Chinese culture. Traditional Chinese Medicine creates a sense of connectedness with Chinese heritage and identity, representing linkages with the past, identity in the present, and continuity for future generations. Underneath the principles and use of Traditional Chinese Medicine there is the pride in the continuous and lengthy history of Chinese culture, and in Traditional Chinese Medicine as a core part of that culture – a cultural achievement. Traditional Chinese Medicine is perceived as a symbol of Chinese identity, both as the source and the product of culture.

For the participants in the studies in this book, the quest for self-understanding and reflectiveness is a creative process. There is a constant struggle to locate self within this changing modern world, and to define social relations with others. Physical identities, ethnic identity, and the search for truth in spiritual dimensions are all post-modern preoccupations. Through the social interactions involving Traditional Chinese Medicine, social acceptance, a sense of belonging and attainment, and a sense of permanence and stability are all made possible.

Another crucial element of Chinese identity is the relationship between Traditional Chinese Medicine and food, both of which are important in Chinese culture. Food cements social relationships including the crucial mother–child reciprocal bond, which is nurtured through the giving and taking Traditional Chinese Medicine. Likewise, Traditional Chinese Medicine is involved in cementing friendships and promoting the role of reproduction. Traditional Chinese Medicine as food is also used to develop the physical body for the social environment, where physical appearances are valued.

Finally, Traditional Chinese Medicine as food is used for preventive purposes and contributes to promoting good health, because Traditional Chinese Medicine philosophy is rooted in preventing disease and self-care.

Balance

Balance in *yin* and *yang* emphasises co-existence, dynamic change without fixing one's ideas, and mutual acceptance in spite of differences. Traditional Chinese Medicine and Western medicine are both fundamentally different and complementary in nature. The difference between these two medical models resides in the concept of 'wholeness' and the interconnectedness of each part to the whole. Traditional Chinese Medicine embraces the holistic approach to people and their connections with the environment: 'the oneness of humans with the universe'. Balance and harmony in life are also key components in the philosophies of living that seek to define all human relationships.

Through Traditional Chinese Medicine, Chinese people in Australia, Mainland China, Taiwan, Hong Kong, Macau and elsewhere experience a strong sense of Chinese identity, a sense of belonging, and a will to transmit Chinese culture.

Finally, I believe that the traditional Chinese philosophies and the cultural values that are presented in this book to underpin Traditional Chinese Medicine offer some solutions to this unsettled modern world. The human dimension of self-cultivation and social interaction, let me repeat, are expressed by trying to do one's very best in life, caring for and being considerate toward others, filial piety, mutual respect and trust, harmony and balance, co-existence and accepting differences. These are all positive attributes which, when applied with our whole hearts, are truly humanistic.

References

Adams J, Sibbritt D, Easthope G and Young A (2003) The profile of women who consult alternative health practitioners in Australia, *Medical Journal Australia* 179(15): 297–300.

Akerlind G (2002) Principles and practice in phenomenographic research, *Proceeding of the International Symposium on Current Issues in Phenomenography*, held in Canberra Australia.

Analects, a book in the Confucian Canon (c. 400 BCE). Trans. J Legge (1893), reprinted as *Confucian Analects, The Great Learning and The Doctrine of the Mean* (1998). SMC Publishing, Taipei.

Anderson E (1988) *The Food of China*. Yale University Press, New Haven and London.

Andrews B (1996) Tailoring Tradition: the impact of modern medicine in traditional Chinese Medicine, 1887-1937. PhD thesis, Cambridge University, accessed at http://www.ucl.ac.uk/histmed/PDFS/Teaching/MA/chinese/C123-Lecture9.pdf on 14 July 2007.

Australian Bureau of Statistics (2001) *People Speaking Chinese Languages, Sydney: A Social Atlas*. AGPS, Canberra.

Australian Bureau of Statistics (2006) 'Complementary health therapists' in *Australian and New Zealand Standard Classification of Occupations* 1st Ed. AGPS, Canberra.

Bary W and Bloom I (1999) *Sources of Chinese Tradition*. Columbia University Press, New York.

Bauman Z (1992) *Intimations of Postmodernity*. Routledge, London.

Baynes C (Ed.) (1965) *The I Ching*. Routledge and Kegan Paul, London.

Beinfield H and Korngold E (1991) *Between Heaven and Earth*. Ballantine Publishing Group, New York.

Bennis W (2003) *On becoming a leader: The leadership classic*. Basic Books, New York.

Bensoussan A, Myers S and Carlton A (2000) Risks associated with the practice of traditional Chinese medicine – An Australian study, *Archives of Family Medicine* 9(10): 1071–1078.

Bensoussan A, Myers S, Drew A, Whyte I and Dawson A (2002) Development of a Chinese herbal medicine toxicology database, *Journal of Toxicology: Clinical Toxicology*, 40(i2): 159–168.

Blair B (1995) *Healing Traditions: Alternative Medicine and the Healing Professions*. University of Pennsylvania Press, Philadelphia.

Bocock R (1993) *Consumption*. Routledge, London.

Bourdieu P (1984) *Distinction*. Harvard University Press, Cambridge.

Bowers J and Purcel E (Eds) (1974) *Medicine and Societies in China*. Josiah Macy Jr Foundation, New York.

Brah A (1996) *Cartographies of Diaspora: Contesting Identities*. Routledge, London.

C&SD, HKSAR (2000) *Thematic Household Survey Report No. 3*. Census and Statistics Department, Hong Kong.

Cash T (1990) The psychology of physical appearance: aesthetics, attitudes and images, in F Cash and T Pruzinsky (Eds), *Body Image*, pp. 51–79. Guilford, New York,.

Chaliand G and Rageau J (1995) *The Penguin Atlas of Diasporas*. Viking, New York.

Chan M, Mok E, Wong Y, Tong T, Day M, Tang C and Wong D (2003) 'Attitudes of Hong Kong Chinese to traditional Chinese medicine and Western medicine: survey and cluster analysis', *Complementary Therapies in Medicine*, 11 (2): 103–109.

Chan Y (1994) *Chinese Culture: A conversation* (in Chinese). Joint Publishing, Hong Kong.

Chia R, Allred L and Jerzak P (1997) 'Attitudes toward women in Taiwan and China', *Psychology of Women Quarterly* 21: 137–150.

Choice (2001) 'Alternative therapies: do they help?' *Australian Consumers' Association*, September: 1.

Chow S (2005) *Ji Du Zhou Yi (I Ching: an analysis and reading)* 3rd Ed. (in Chinese). Century Publishing, Shanghai.

Chun A (1996) 'Discourses of Identity in the Changing Spaces of Public Culture in Taiwan, Hong Kong and Singapore', *Theory, Culture and Society* 13(1): 51–75.

Chu LC and Wong PS (Eds) (2003) 'On Levelling All Things' in *Chuang Tzu* (in Chinese). King Na University, Guangzhou.

Chung L (Ed) (2004) *Lao Tzu* (in Chinese). Harbin publishing, Harbin.

Classic of Filial Piety (722 CE) Trans. J Legge (1889), reprinted in *The Sacred Books of the East: The Texts of Confucianism*, Vol.III Part I: *The Shu King, the Religions Portions of the Shih King, the Hsiao King* (722CE), pp. 465–486. Clarendon Press, Oxford.

Cleary C (1993) (trans. and presented), *The Essential Taoism: Initiation into the heart of Taoism through the authentic Tao Te Ching and the inner teaching of Chuang Tzu*. Castle Books, New Jersey.

Connell R (2002) *Gender*. Polity Press, Cambridge.

Cooley C (1926) 'The roots of social knowledge', *The American Journal of Sociology* 32(7): 59–71.

Coward R (1983) *Patriarchal Precedents*. Routledge and Kegan Paul, London.

Creel H (1975) *Chinese Thought from Confucius to Mao Tse-tung*. The University of Chicago Press, Chicago.

Curtis S and Taket A (1996) *Health and Societies: Changing Perspectives*. Edward Arnold, London.

Dawson M (1995) *The Conduct of Life*. Carlton House, New York.

DSEC (2004) *Macau Health Statistics*, Statistics and Census Services, DSEC, Macau.

Djao W (2003) *Being Chinese: Voices from the Diaspora*. University of Arizona Press, Arizona.

Duhl L (1981) The social context of health, in A Hastings, J Fadiman and J Gordon (Eds), *Health for the Whole Person*, pp. 43–55. Bantam Books, Toronto.

Edensor T (2002) *National Identity, Popular Culture and Everyday Life*. Berg, Oxford.

Eisenberg D, Davis R, Ettner S, Appel S, Wilkey S, Rompay M and Kessler R (1998) Trends in alternative medicine use in the United States, 1990–1997, *Journal of the American Medical Association* 280: 1569–1575.

Ell K and Castaneda I (1998) 'Health care seeking behaviour', in S Loue (Ed), *Handbook of Immigrant Health*, pp.125–143. Pleuna Press, New York.

Erikson E (1968) *Identity: Youth and Crisis*. Faber and Faber, London.

Fitzpatrick R (1984) 'Lay concepts of illness', in R Fitzpatrick, J Hinton, S Newman, G Scrambler and J Thompson (Eds), *The Experience of Illness*, pp.11–31.Tavistock Publications, London.

Fitzpatrick R, Hinton J, Newman J, Scrambler G and Thompson C (Eds) (1984) *The Experiences of Illness*. Tavistock Publications, London.

Flaws B (1994) *Imperial Secrets of Health and Longevity*. Blue Poppy Press, Boulder.

Foucault M (1986) *The Care of the Self, The History of Sexuality Vol. III*. Penguin Books, London.

Foucault M (1988) 'Technologies of the Self', in P Hutton (Ed), *Technologies of the Self*, pp.16–49. University of Massachusetts Press, Massachusetts.

Foucault M (1990) *The Will to Knowledge, the History of Sexuality Vol.1*. Penguin Books, London.

Fu LS (1975) *Chinese History* Vol 1. Po Wen Books, Hong Kong.

Fung YL (1948) *A Short History of Chinese Philosophy*. Trans. D Bodde. Macmillan, London.

Fung YL (1973) *A Short History of Chinese Philosophy*. Trans. D Bodde. Free Press, New York.

Fung YL (1983) *A History of Chinese Philosophy: The Period of the Philosophers* Vol. 1. Trans. D Bodde. Princeton University Press, Princeton.

Furnham A (1988) *Lay theories: Everyday Understanding of Problems in the Social Sciences*. Pergamon Press, Oxford.

Furnham A (1994) Explaining health and illness: lay perceptions on current and future health, the causes of illness, and the nature of recovery. *Social Science and Medicine* 39(5): 715–725.

Furth C (1987) Concepts of pregnancy, childbirth, and infancy in Ching Dynasty China, *Journal of Asian Studies* 46(1): 7–35.

Gabardi W (2001) *Negotiating Postmodernism*. University of Minnesota Press, Minneapolis.

Geertz C (1975) *The Interpretation of Cultures*. Hutchinson, London.

Gerber R (1992) Phenomenography as an important qualitative approach to research in Geography. *Paper presented to the International Geographical Union Symposium on Geographical Education*, Boulder, Colorado, August 3–7.

Gerber R (1996) 'Interpretive approaches to geographical and environmental education', in M William (Ed), *Understanding geographical and environmental education: The role of research*, pp.12–25. Cassell, London.

Gerber R (2005) Personal communication.

Giddens A (1991) *Modernity and Self-Identity*. Polity Press, Cambridge.

Goffman E (1959) *Presentation of Self in Everyday Life*. Penguin Books, London.

Goffman E (1963) *Stigma: Notes on the Management of Spoiled Identity*. Simon and Schuster, New York.

Gorden C (Ed.) (1980) *Michel Foucault: Power/knowledge*. Harvester, Brighton.

Gorey J, Wahlqvist M and Boyce N (1992) Adverse reaction to a Chinese herbal remedy, *Medical Journal Australia* 157: 484–486.

Greg S (1996) Binary opposition and sexual power in Paradise Lost, *The Midwest Quarterly* 37(4): 383–390.

Guo Z (2000) *Ginseng and Aspirin*. Cornell University Press, Ithaca and London.

Hage B, Tang K, Li R, Lin V, Chow T and Thien F (2001) A qualitative investigation into the use of health services among Melbourne Chinese, *Australian Journal of Primary Health* 7(2): 38–40.

Hammer L (1990) *Dragon Rises Red Bird Flies*. Station Hill Press, New York.

Harmsworth K and Lewith G (2001) Attitude to traditional Chinese medicine amongst Western trained doctors in the People's Republic of China, *Social Science and Medicine* 52: 149–153.

Hawkes T (1972) *Metaphor*. Methuen, London.

Heider J (1985) *The Tao of leadership: Lao Tzu's Tao Te Ching*. Humanics New Age, Atlanta, Georgia.

Hermitary (2002) *Tao Chien (Tao Yuan-ming) Poet of Reclusion,* accessed at www.hermitary.com/articles/tao_chien.html on 16 July 2007.

Ho D (1989) Continuity and variation in Chinese patterns of socialisation, *Journal of Marriage and the Family* 51(1): 149–163.

Ho P and Lisowski F (1993) *Concepts of Chinese Science and Traditional Healing Arts: A Historical Review*. World Scientific Publishing, Singapore.

Holbrook B (1977) The Social-Structural and Theoretical Bases of Chinese Psycho-Social Medicine: Disciplinal Kinship and the Transformation of Culture into Flesh. PhD thesis, Yale University, Connecticut.

Howson A (2004) *The Body in Society: An Introduction*. Polity, Cambridge.

Hui CW (1994) *Development of Chinese Culture* (in Chinese). Chinese University Press, Taipei.

Hutton P (1988) 'Foucault, Freud, and the technologies of the self', in L Martin, H Gutman and P Hutton (Eds), *Technologies of the Self: A Seminar with Michel Foucault*, pp.121–140. University of Massachusetts Press, Massachusetts.

Jewell J (1982) 'Theoretical basis of Chinese Traditional Medicine', in S Hillier and J Jewell (Eds), *Health Care and Traditional Medicine in China, 1900–1982*, pp.221–241. Routledge and Kegan Paul, London.

Johnson M (Ed.) (1981) *Philosophical Perspectives on Metaphor*. University of Minnesota Press, Minneapolis.

Jones R and Vincent A (1998) Can we tame wild medicine? *New Scientist* 3(Jan): 27–29.

Kao Tsze, a book in the works of *Mencius* (c. 371–289 BCE). Trans. W Dobson (1963). Oxford University Press, London.

Keffer D (2001) *Outlaws of the Marsh: A somewhat less than critical commentary history of the novel*. Foreign Language Press, Beijing.

Kelen B (1983) *Confucius*. Graham Brash, Singapore.

Khng C (2003) Trends in the utilisation of traditional Chinese medicine in rural China: a case study of Yuhang County, Zhejiang. PhD thesis, University of Guelph, Canada.

King Hui of Liang, a book in the works of *Mencius* (c. 371–289 BCE). Trans. DC Lau (1970). Penguin Classics, London.

Kleinman A (1978) 'Culture illness and cure'. *Annuals of Internal Medicine* 88: 251–259.

Kleinman A and Seeman D (2000) 'Personal experience of illness', in G Albrecht, R Fitzpatrick and S Scrimshaw (Eds), *Handbook of Social Studies In Health and Medicine*, pp.230–242. Sage Publications, London.

Knight Ridder Tribune Business News (2006) 'Out with Chinese medicine' (Editorial), 29 November: 1. Washington.

Kung-sun Chau, a book in the works of *Mencius* (c. 371–289 BCE). Trans. W Dobson (1963). Oxford, London.

Lakoff G and Johnson M (1980) *Metaphors We Live By*. University of Chicago Press, Chicago.

Lam K and Wong Y (1995) *Discourses of Chinese Culture* (in Chinese). Mei Ah Publishing, Hong Kong.

Lam KY (1995) 'The characteristics of Chinese culture', in KY Lam and YS Wong (Eds), *Chinese Culture* (in Chinese), pp.6–10. Hong Kong Educational Books, Hong Kong.

Larson L (1977) *Major Themes in Sociological Theory*. David McKay Company, Boston.

Last J (1963) The Iceberg: Completing the clinical picture in general practice, *The Lancet* 2: 28–31.

Lau T (1978) *The Development of Chinese Literature* (in Chinese). Hock Lum, Hong Kong.

Lee L (1991) 'On the margins of the Chinese discourse: some personal thoughts on the cultural meaning of the periphery', in W Tu (Ed), *The Living Tree: The Changing Meaning of Being Chinese Today*, pp.221–241. Stanford University Press, California.

Lee R (1980) Perceptions and uses of Chinese medicine among the Chinese in Hong Kong, *Culture, Medicine, Psychiatry* 4: 345–375.

Legge J (1998) *The Chinese Classics*, reprinted (1998) a reprint of the original (1891). SMC Publishing Inc, Taipei.

Leung B and Gerber R (2006) 'Conceptions of Leadership in Traditional Chinese Medicine by the Chinese People in Macau and Hong Kong', paper presented at the *National Medicine Symposium on Quality Care of Medicine*, Canberra, 7–9 June.

Leung B (2004) Traditional Chinese Medicine in the Chinese diaspora, Australia: a social analysis. PhD thesis, University of New England, Armidale NSW.

Leung S (1989) *The Main Concepts of Chinese Culture* (in Chinese). Joint Publishing, Hong Kong.

Leung S (1994) *The Essence of Chinese Culture* (in Chinese). Joint Publishing, Hong Kong.

Leung Y (1995) *The Search in History and Reflections on Culture* (in Chinese). Hong Kong Education Books, Hong Kong.

Lin A and Flaws B (1991) *The Dao of Increasing Longevity and Conserving One's Life*. Blue Poppy Press, Boulder.

Li Lou, a book in the works of *Mencius* (c. 371–289 BCE) Trans. DC Lau (1970). Penguin Classics, London.

Lin Y (1977) *My Country and My People*, Heinemann Educational Books (Asia), Hong Kong.

Lin Y (1938) *The Importance of Living*. William Heinemann, London.

Liu J (2000) 'Chinese medicine no threat to nature'. *China Daily* (North American Ed.), January 10: 8. New York.

Liu WJ (2006) *The Future of Traditional Chinese Medicine in China*, APSI Research Project. Beijing, China, accessed at http://www.duke.edu/APSI/grants/Summer06StudentReports/WenjingLiu.doc on 17 June 2007.

Ludman E, Newman J and Lynn L (1989) Blood-building foods in contemporary Chinese populations, *Journal of the American Dietetic Association* 89(8): 1122–1125.

Lupton D (1994) *Medicine as Culture*. Sage Publications, London.

M2 Presswire (2006) 'Defra: call for UK China partnerships to find traditional medicine alternatives', 25 July: 1. M2 Communications, Coventry.

Malinowski B (1963) *Sex, Culture, and Myth*. Rupert Hart-Davis, London.

Marton F (1981) Phenomenography in describing conceptions of the world around us, *Instructional Science* 10: 177–200.

Marton F (1986) Phenomenography: a research approach to investigating different understandings of reality, *Journal of Thought* 21(3): 28–49.

Mau TS (1988) 'Characteristics of Chinese culture', in YS Chow (Ed.), *Reconstruction of Traditional Culture* (in Chinese), pp. 3–34. Daily Cultural Publishing, Taipei.

Mau TS (2005) *Nineteen Lectures on Chinese Culture* (in Chinese). Shanghai Century Publishing, Shanghai.

Mechanic D (1992) Health and illness behaviour and patient-practitioner relationships, *Social Science and Medicine* 34(12):1345–1350.

Mencius (c. 371–289 BCE). Trans. W. Dobson (1963). Oxford University Press, London.

Mingpao (2003, 1 October) Newspaper (in Chinese). Hong Kong.

Morris D (1998) *Illness and Culture in the Postmodern Age*. University of California Press, Berkeley.

Muller F (Ed.) (1966) *Sacred Books of the East*. Motilal Banarsidass, Delhi.

Needham, J (1974) *Science and Civilisation in China Vol 2: History of Scientific Thought*. Cambridge University Press, Cambridge.

Needham J (1983) *Science and Civilisation in China: Vol. 5: Chemistry and Chemical Technology*. Cambridge University Press, Cambridge.

Nei Jing (*Yellow Emperor's Canon of Internal Medicine*) (Tang Dynasty 618–907 CE) Trans. N Wu and A Wu (1999). Chinese Science and Technology Press, Beijing.

Nettleton S (1995) *The Sociology of Health and Illness*. Polity Press, Cambridge.

Ng T, Chan Y and Yu Y (1991) Encephalopathy and neuropathy following ingestion of Chinese herbal broth containing podophyllin, *Journal Neurological Science* 101: 107–113.

Pang E, Jordan-March M, Silverstein M and Cody M (2003), Health-seeking behaviours of elderly Chinese Americans: shifts in expectations, *The Gerontologist* 43(6): 864–874.

Pawluch D, Cain R and Gillett J (2000) Lay constructions of HIV and complementary therapy use, *Social Science and Medicine* 51: 251–264.

Pearce F (2001) Greater than the parts: how does Traditional Chinese Medicine compare with Western treatments? *New Scientist* 26(May): 51–53.

Penny B (1993) 'Qigong, Daoism and science: some contexts for the Qigong boom', in M Lee and A Syrokomka-Stefanowska (Eds), *Modernisation of the Chinese Past*, p.176. Wild Peony, Broadway NSW.

Pillsbury B (1978) 'Doing the Month': Confinement and convalescence of Chinese women after childbirth, *Social Science and Medicine* 12(1B): 11–22.

Plain Questions, a part of the *Nei Jing* (*Yellow Emperor's Canon of Internal Medicine*) (Tang Dynasty 618–907 CE). Trans. N Wu and A Wu (1999). Chinese Science and Technology Press, Beijing.

Plummer D (1999) *One of the Boys*. Harrington Park Press, Binghamton.

Pong P (1992) 'The humanistic spirit in Chinese culture', in CY Cheung and YW Wong (Eds), *The Reassessment of Traditional Chinese Culture* (in Chinese) Vol 1, pp. 56–63. The Commercial Press, Hong Kong.

Porkert M and Ullmann C (1982) *Chinese Medicine*. William Morrow, New York.

Prior L, Pang C and Huat S (2000) Beliefs and accounts of illness: views from two Cantonese speaking communities in England, *Sociology of Health and Illness* 22(6): 815–839.

Qian M (1979) *Chinese culture and Chinese Racial Characteristics: A Historical Perspective* (in Chinese). Chinese University of Hong Kong, Hong Kong.

Qian M (2004) *Soul and Heart* (in Chinese). Keilin, Normal University Press, Quangxi.

Rabinow P (Ed.) (1994) *Michael Foucault Ethics: Subjectivity and truth.* The New Press, New York.

Reid D (1996) *Traditional Chinese Medicine.* Shambhala, Boston.

Riesman D (1963) *The Lonely Crowd.* Yale University Press, Connecticut.

Ruan F (1991) *Sex in China.* Plenum Press, New York.

Sandberg J (1997) Are phenomenographic results reliable?, *Higher Education Research and Development* 16(2): 203–212.

Sarup M (1996) *Identity, Culture and the Postmodern World.* Edinburgh University Press, Edinburgh.

Schipper K (1993) *The Taoist Body.* University of California Press, Berkeley.

Shen Y (2001) *Dragon Seed in the Antipodes.* Melbourne University Press, Melbourne.

Shi L (1995) 'Traditional remedies heal the world', *China Daily, 23 June, p. 9.2.*

Shilling C (1993) *The Body and Social Theory.* Sage Publications, London.

Shils E (1981) *Tradition.* Faber and Faber, London.

Siahpush M (1999) Postmodern attitudes about health: a population-based exploratory study, *Complementary Therapies in Medicine* 7: 164–169.

Siegel R (1979) Ginseng abuse syndrome – problems with the panacea, *Journal of American Medical Association* 241: 1614–1615.

Sivin N (2003) *Science and Medicine in Chinese History,* accessed at http://ccat.sas.upenn.edu/~nsivin/ropp.html on 17 Jun 2007.

Smith A, Kellett E and Schmerlaib Y (1998) *The Australian Guide to Healthy Eating.* Commonwealth Department of Health and Family Services, Victoria.

Spiritual Pivot, a part of the *Nei Jing* (*Yellow Emperor's Canon of Internal Medicine*) (Tang Dynasty 618–907 CE). Trans. N Wu and A Wu (1999). Chinese Science and Technology Press, Beijing.

Stacey J (1983) *Patriarchy and Socialist Revolution in China.* University of California Press, Berkeley.

Stanford Encyclopedia of Philosophy (2007) *Mohism,* accessed at http://plato.stanford.edu/entries/mohism/ on 17 June 2007.

Straten N and Koeppen G (1983) *Concept of Health, Disease and Vitality in Traditional Chinese Society: A Psychological Interpretation.* Steiner, Wiesbaden.

Svensson L (1997) Theoretical foundations of phenomenography, *Higher Education Research and Development* 16(2): 159–171.

Sun G (1988) *Health Preservation and Rehabilitation.* Shanghai College of Traditional Chinese Medicine Press, Shanghai.

Sun LK (2004) *Deep Structure of Chinese Culture* (in Chinese). Guangxi Normal University Press, Keilin.

Sun YS (1963) *San Min Chui I: The Three Principles of the People* (from a series of his lectures in 1924 with two supplementary chapters by Chiang Kai-shek), trans. FW Price. China Publishing Co, Taipei.

Sun ZY (1999) On Mohist Humanism and Scientific of Spirit, *Philosophical Forum* (in Chinese) 28: 4–23.

Tang CI (2000) *Spiritual Value of Chinese Culture* (in Chinese). Ching Chung, Taipei.

Tang OS (Ed.) (2005) *Interesting quotations of I Ching* (in Chinese). Hoi Pei, Bai Hua Literature and Art Publishing House, Tianjin.

Tang K and Easthope G (2000) What constitutes treatment effectiveness? The differential judgements of Chinese Australian patients and doctors, *Complementary Therapies in Medicine* 8(4): 241–247.

Tang Wan Kung, a book in the works of *Mencius* (c. 371–289 BCE). Trans. J Legge (1893), reprinted as *Mencius* (1998). SMC Publishing, Taipei.

Tao Te Ching (600–400 BCE) Trans. D Lau (1963). Penguin Books, London.

Tao MP (2005) *The Passion of Peach Flower Land: The Work of Tao Yuen Ming.* The Way International Cultural Ltd, Taipei.

The Analects or *Lun Yu* (year unknown) 18 Languages CD-ROM. Confucius Publishing, Vancouver.

The Doctrine of the Mean, a book in the Confucian Canon (c. 400 BCE) Trans. J Legge (1893), reprinted as *Confucian Analects, The Great Learning and The Doctrine of the Mean* (1998). SMC Publishing, Taipei.

The Great Learning, a book in the Confucian Canon (c. 400 BCE) Trans. J Legge (1893), reprinted as *Confucian Analects, The Great Learning and The Doctrine of the Mean* (1998). SMC Publishing, Taipei.

Thompson C and Hirschman E (1995) Understanding the socialised body: a poststructuralist analysis of consumers' self-care practices, *Journal of Consumer Research* 22(2): 139–154.

Tsin Sin, a book in the works of *Mencius* (c. 371–289 BCE). Trans. W Dobson (1963). Oxford University Press, London.

Tsao H (c. 1717–1763) *Dream of the Red Chamber,* with a continuation by Kao Ou. Trans. Wang C (1983). G Brash, Singapore.

Tu W (Ed.) (1991) *The Living Tree: The Changing Meaning of Being Chinese Today.* Stanford University Press, California.

Unschuld P (1985) *Medicine in China: A History of Ideas.* University of California Press, Berkeley.

Vanherweghem J, Depierreux M and Tielemans C (1993) Rapidly progressive interstitial renal fibrosis in young women: Association with slimming regimen including Chinese herbs, *The Lancet* 341: 387–391.

Victoria Ministerial Advisory Committee (1998) *Traditional Chinese Medicine: Report on Options for Regulation of Practitioners.* Victoria Government of Human Services, Melbourne.

Wai C (1995) *Chinese Culture* (in Chinese). Buffalo, Taipei.

Weber M (1951) *The Religion of China.* Free Press, Illinois.

Wikipedia Encyclopedia. *John G. Kerr,* accessed at http://en.wikipedia.org/wiki/John_G._Kerr on 17 June 2007.

Wimmer A and Schiller N (2003) Methodological nationalism, the social sciences, and the study of migration: an essay in historical epistemology, *International Migration Review* 37(i3): 576–611.

Wong YL (1995) 'The ideal character in traditional Chinese', in KY Lam and YS Wong (Eds), *Chinese Culture* (in Chinese), pp.78–79. Hong Kong Educational Books, Hong Kong.

Wright M (1959) *The Sociological Imagination*. Oxford University Press, New York.

Wu D (1991) 'The construction of Chinese and non-Chinese identities', in W Tu (Ed), *The Living Tree: The Changing Meaning of Being Chinese Today*, pp.148–166. Stanford University Press, California.

Xinhua News (2001) 'China, Australia cooperate in developing Traditional Chinese Medicine', 19 April: 1008.

Xu X (2001) *Principles of Traditional Chinese Medicine*. YMAA Publications, Boston.

Yan HK (1988) 'Reestablishment of morality', in YS Chow (Ed), *The Reestablishment of Traditional Chinese Culture*, pp.73–116. Time Publishing, Taipei.

Yeung H (2004) *Book of the Means, The Great Learning: Notes* (in Chinese). The Country Publisher, Taipei.

Yiu W (1984) *The Chinese Strategies for Healthy Living* (in Chinese). Man Jing Publishing, Taipei.

Yu S (1994) *The Modern Interpretation of Traditional Chinese Thinking* (in Chinese). Luen King, Taipei.

Zhang Y and Rose K (1999) *Who Can Ride the Dragon? An Explanation of the Cultural Roots of Traditional Chinese Medicine*. Paradigm Publications, Massachusetts.

Chinese Dynasties

中國朝代表

Note: BCE indicates 'Before Current Era', and CE indicates 'Current Era'.

Dynasty 朝代	Time Period 時期
Shang 商	1700–1122 BCE
Zhou 周	1122–221 BCE
Spring and Autumn Period 春秋時代	770–470 BCE
Warring States Period 戰國時代	475–221 BCE
Qin 秦	221–207 BCE
Han 漢	206 BCE – 220 CE
Wai 魏, **Jin** 晉, **Nan-bei Chai** 南北朝	220–581 CE
Sui 隋	581–618 CE
Tang 唐	618–907 CE
Five Dynasties 五代十國	907–979 CE
Song 宋	960–1279 CE
Yuan 元	1279–1368 CE
Ming 明	1368–1644 CE
Qing 清	1644–1911 CE
Republic of China 中華民國	1912–1949 CE
People's Republic of China 中華人民共和國	1949 CE –

Chinese Classic Literature and Philosophers

I Ching or *The Book of Changes* 易經 (3000–4000 BCE) – One of the oldest surviving Chinese classics, *I Ching* is a metaphysical treatise of both cosmic and moral order, based on *yin* and *yang*. Sixty-four hexagrams, graphic images consisting of six solid or broken lines arranged vertically, are used to explain change phenomenon and relationships with other signs. The solid line in the hexagrams (—) represents *yang* (heaven) and the broken line (– –) represents *yin* (the earth). According to *I Ching*, reality is understood as being constantly changing and dynamic, and nothing is absolute.

Sheung Shu 尚書 (2300–1000 BCE) – The oldest Chinese historical book, *Sheung Shu* recorded events of the Yu, Hsia, Shang and Zhou dynasties.

Book of Odes / Shijing 詩經 (early Zhou dynasty, around 1122–570 BCE) – The earliest work of Chinese poems and literature, *Shijing* contained a compilation of 305 poems, court festival songs, sacrifices for gods and ancestral spirits, dynastic legends, and tales of love and war, many combined with music and dancing. The poems described the turbulent events of 500 years, reflecting the realities of life for the people in those times. A famous saying of Confucius, 'Having no depraved thought', was attributed to *Shijing*.

Book of Rites / Li Ki 禮記 (800–500 BCE) – This book recorded Chinese religious practices and the social forms and ceremonies of the times.

Zuo Zhuan 左傳 (722–468 BCE) – The earliest work of narrative history (author unknown), *Zuo Zhuan* serves as a bridge linking *Sheung Shu* and *Historical Record*. In *Zuo Zhuan* was given a realistic account of the people and events of the Spring and Autumn Period. The perspective employed to give meaning to the turmoils experienced during this era was based on Confucian principles such as 'the virtuous will win and the evil will be punished'.

Lao Tzu 老子 (600–400 BCE) – Lao Tzu was the father of Taoism, the first thinker in the Chinese and Western histories to advance the idea that all phenomena on earth come from nature (*Tao Te Ching*, Chapter 25). The cosmological vision of Tao's nature operates in an endless, spontaneous circular manner, and phenomena are relative and relational. His central ideas consisted of valuing self, loving and preserving life (he believed that one's life was in one's hands and there was always something one could do about it), avoiding extremes (the use of the middle way), *wuwei* (doing less), and harmony with nature. His ideas are expounded in *Tao Te Ching* and in some chapters of *Chuang Tzu*, the work of Chuang Tzu (399–295 BCE), a keen Tao philosopher. Lao Tzu's date of birth was unknown, some saying it was between 600–300 BCE and others around 600 BCE. However, historian Fung Yu-lan (1948) suggested Lao Tzu probably lived between the time of Mozi (479–381 BCE) and Mencius (371–289 BCE); Mencius mentioned Lao Tzu as 'influential' in his text, but Mozi did not mention Lao Tzu.

Tao Te Ching 道德經 (600–400 BCE) – This book, attributed to Lao Tzu, consisted of 5000 words. The aim of the book was to help people to find a way of life through the difficulties of the times. Tao, the Way, was perceived as the origin of the universe as well as a method for maintaining harmony between individuals and in the world. All things were seen as being made up of *yin* and *yang*, and the blending of the two forces was seen to produce *qi*. The non-dualistic relationships of naturalness, equal standing and balance in the life-world and the non-judgemental attitude of *wuwei* (non-action) permeated the text of *Tao Te Ching*.

Confucius 孔夫子 (c. 551–479 BCE) – Confucius has been regarded by the Chinese as a great thinker, social philosopher and teacher, and as China's first private teacher. Confucius attracted many followers and is believed to have had 3000 disciples, among them 70 who themselves became distinguished. Confucius's philosophy embraces personal and social relationships and governmental ideals. One of Confucius's cardinal teachings, *yen* (benevolence), embraces the total moral standard of a person, including the moral quality of one's thoughts. Confucius believed that physical and mental strengths were constituted in the social dimension; one cultivates the self by applying one's strength and commitment in human relationships. He taught that love is not equal in relationships but that there are degrees of love.

Mozi 墨子 (468–376 BCE) – Little is know of the life of Mozi (also Mo Tzu), the founder of the school of Mohism who lived between the times of Confucius and Mencius. He was the first Chinese philosopher to point out the drawbacks of traditional Chinese ideas and the first to oppose the teachings of Confucius. Whereas Confucius admired and justified ancient civilisation and tradition, Mozi opposed traditional attitudes and practices. Where Confucius taught 'benevolence' as a 'degree of love', Mozi's central teaching was 'universal love'. Mozi's also emphasised equality, that is, people in a group should all 'enjoy equally and suffer equally'.

Mohist Doctrines 墨學教條 (468–376 BCE) – A collection of the doctrine and writings of Mozi (468–376 BCE) and his followers, a number of the 53 chapters were devoted to the principle of universal love. A distinguishing feature of Mozi's doctrine was the emphasis on 'benefit' 利, that is, doing something good for the country and the people. This doctrine set the general standard in humanism. Mozi's central ideas were encapsulated in the Ten Theses: (1) elevating the worthy; (2) exalting unity; (3) all embracing love; (4) against military and aggression; (5) frugality of expenditure; (6) frugality of funerals; (7) heaven's will; (8) elucidating the spirit; (9) against music; (10) against fatalism.

Mencius 孟子 (c. 371–289 BCE) – Mencius defended the teachings of Confucius and developed and added greater depth to Confucianism, earning Mencius the title of Second Sage after Confucius. Mencius held that all human nature is essentially good. Significantly, he added a deeper moral dimension to the role of the 'heart', saying that one 'thinks' with the heart. Mencius applied the concept of 'benevolence' more specifically than Confucius, referring to the relationships between parent and child and, by extension, to the ruler's virtue and responsibilities toward the people. In his political philosophy, Mencius emphasised supremacy of the people and the requirement for government to be benevolent.

Confucian Canon / The Four Books of Confucianism 四書 (c. 400 BCE and later) –

The Great Learning 大學 – A Chinese classic handed down by the Confucian school, *The Great Learning* illustrates the importance of acquiring knowledge about virtue as a prime requisite for the ancient learner.

The Doctrine of the Mean / Chung Yung 中庸 – Attributed to Confucius's grandson, Tsze Sze, the 33 chapters of this book describe how to obtain perfect virtue. *Chung* means 'in the middle' or 'equilibrium' and *yung* means 'common or ordinary' or 'harmony'. Emotions such as pleasure, anger, sorrow, or joy, if not expressed, are viewed as the state of 'equilibrium'; if expressed in the proper manner without extremes, they are called 'harmony'.

Analects 論語 – A collection of sayings attributed to Confucius, the *Analects* were complied by his disciples around 481–221 BCE, after Confucius's death. The core theme throughout the *Analects* is *yen* (benevolence/humanity), a 'gradation' or degree of love.

Mencius / The Works of Mencius 孟子 – These seven books (each of two parts) collect the work of Mencius (c. 371–289 BCE) and his contemporaries: *Liang Hiu Wang* (Book 1), *Gong Sun Chou* (Book 2), *Teng Wen Gong* (Book 3), *Li Lou* (Book 4), *Wan Zhang* (Book 5), *Gaozi* (Book 6), and *Jin Xin* (Book 7). The book titles, taken from the opening sentences in most cases, are the names of people with whom Mencius had conversations. Mencius's ideas basically followed and expanded on the teachings of Confucius. Central to Mencius's doctrine is the thesis that human nature is essentially good, based on the humanistic understanding of Heaven, humanity, harmony, and self-cultivation.

Chuang Tzu 莊子 (399–295 BCE) – Considered the greatest of the early Taoists and a mystic, little is known about Chuang Tzu's life apart from his writings. He refused to take the conventions of life during his time for granted, and preferred non-government. He developed the Taoist doctrine further with his perspective on the oneness of humans with the universe. His philosophy was encapsulated by 'nature': he advised people to follow nature (what is natural in oneself) in order to achieve happiness. According to Chuang Tzu, what is of nature is internal, and what is of man is external. Therefore, following nature was the way to attain happiness, and following man was the way to misery. Chuang Tzu's writings were highly praised for his lively and vivid style and the use of simple devices such as birds, fish, trees and carpenters to describe people's lives. His writings contained transcendental elements, 'to transcend what is real, what is wise and what is happy', in which the real and not-real were fused together. Transcending time and space, life and death were also fused, based on the conception of the unity of human and universe.

Sze-ma Tsien 司馬遷 (145–? BCE) – Sze-ma Tsien is considered the father of Chinese historiography. Sze-ma Tsien's father, an official historian, had entrusted Sze-ma Tsien with the responsibility of writing an historical book. At the age of 42, Sze-ma Tsien tried to defend a defeated general and exasperated the king. He was sent to prison and endured the most humiliating punishment of castration. In a moving letter to his friend, he expressed his poignant pain (Lau 1978: 170, my translation):

Every memory engulfs me and tears me apart into pieces. I live restlessly as if defeated; I move around aimlessly as if homeless. The very thought of my humiliation has never failed to bring in flood of tears that wet my clothes.

However, he survived by focussing all his hopes on writing the book and, in spite of his physical and mental torment, spent the rest of his life's energy completing the highly honoured *Historical Record*.

Historical Record 史記 (around 100 BCE) – Compiled by Sze-ma Tsien 司馬遷 and consisting of 130 volumes with a total of 526,500 words, *Historical Record* provided a vivid account of politics, economy, culture, medicine and history, recording from the time of the Yellow Emperor (3rd millennium BCE) until Sze-ma Tsien's own time (Han Dynasty, from 206 BCE until his death).

Tao Yuan-ming 陶淵明 (365–427 CE) – A Chinese poet who wrote 150 poems, Tao Yuan-ming was well known for his poems on nature, notably his garden-and-field poetry in which the harmony between humans and rural settings was displayed. He was well-educated but poor, and declined all jobs offered. He did not care for money or fame and was contented with his lot, finding peace in a simple and humble life as a recluse and farmer. His preference for the spontaneity of nature was reflected in his deeply moving poems of the natural and simple experiences of the people of that time, in which he identified the unity of humans with nature with natural ease, human warmth, humility and simplicity.

Sun Si-miao 孫思邈 (581–682 CE) – A Taoist priest who lived in seclusion during the Tang Dynasty, Sun Si-miao was a great alchemist and medical writer. He was not recognised in his day, but is now well known as the King of Medicine. He studied medicine, gathered herbs, made medicines, and cured people. He wrote many medical treatises including prescriptions and theories, for example, *The Thousand Golden Remedies*. He combined Taoist theories such as *yin* and *yang* and inner virtue with the medical science of hygiene. He provided a code of moral conduct for physicians that all patients should be treated equally and with good conscience. He believed that life was most important, more precious than gold, for a life lost was lost forever. He emphasised the importance of food therapy, and suggested that people could achieve longevity if they adhered to good diet, good emotions, good spirits and good deeds.

Nei Jing / Yellow Emperor's Canon of Internal Medicine 黃帝內經 (Tang Dynasty 618–907 CE) – The authorship of *Nei Jing*, the first Chinese medical classic, is unknown. Appearing to be the work of the legendary Yellow Emperor (3rd Millennium BCE), *Nei Jing* was written in the form of dialogue between the Yellow Emperor and Qibi, a Taoist. The Yellow Emperor raised a series of questions about ways to preserve health and prevent illness. Many chapters were explicitly devoted to the *yin* and *yang* correspondences between man and the environment, providing information on the function of *yin* and *yang* and guidelines for prosperous and declining energies. *Nei Jing* provides an account of human struggle for survival in times of illness during the Spring and Autumn Period and Warring States Period and the subsequent Qin and Han dynasties. A more accurate edition was held to have been compiled by Wang Bing of the Tang dynasty (618–907 CE). *Nei Jing* was comprised of two parts, *Plain Questions* and *Spiritual Pivot*. In the treatise on the Canon and Literature of History (Han Dynasty), *Nei Jing* consisted of 18 rolls, nine in each of *Plain Questions* and *Spiritual Pivot*, but now there are only eight rolls in *Plain Questions*. However Wang Bing noted 81 chapters in each of *Plain Questions* and *Spiritual Pivot* (Wu & Wu 1997).

The Water Margin 水滸傳 (Ming Dynasty, 1368–1644 CE) – The first Chinese novel to be written in vernacular Chinese, *The Water Margin* was written by Shih Nai-an 施耐庵 and edited by Lo Kuan-chung 羅貫中. At first it was divided into 100 chapters and later into 120 chapters. The book depicted the folk art and heroic story of 108 people (105 men and 3 women) who represented various classes of oppressed people. These people were forced to become bandits and retreat to Mount Liang 梁山 (Liang Shan). However, they gathered strength and stood up against power and evil. The story gave vivid accounts of diverse human relationships of love and hate, physical strength and bravery in times of danger, the glory of friendship, and the humanistic spirit of helping the poor. Nowadays, the Chinese saying 'the retreat to Liang Shan' is used to refer to nice people forced into difficult circumstances. (A translation of this novel, *Outlaws of the Marsh*, is available in the commentary by Keffer in 2001, based on the translation by Sidney Shapiro in 1980.)

The Journey to the West 西遊記 (Ming Dynasty, 1368–1644 CE) – The main characters in this supernatural novel written by Wu Cheng-en 吳承恩 included the Monkey 孫悟空, Pigsy 豬八戒, Sandy 沙淨, and a Monk called Hsien Chuag 唐三藏. Many characters in this action-packed novel had super powers, including the central figure of the Monkey, who was depicted as mischievous, humorous and loyal to the Monk, his master. The story related the Monk's journey to the West, meeting many monsters and temptations along the way. The author cleverly used animals to symbolise and criticise people and customs in the real world. Importantly, the novel reflected the courage, loyalty, wit, and positive character of the people. The novel has been very popular among young people for many generations and has been adapted for movies and television shows.

Dream of the Red Chamber 紅樓夢 (Qing Dynasty, 18th Century) – *Dream of the Red Chamber* has been considered the greatest traditional Chinese novel and the first great tragic novel in Chinese literature. Of the novel's 120 chapters, the first 80 were attributed to Tsao Hsueh-chin 曹雪芹 and the last 40 to Kao Ou. The story described a love triangle between three main characters, Jia Bao-yu 賈寶玉, Lin Dai-yu 林黛玉 and Xue Bao-chai 薛寶釵, the victims of feudal society. The novel, a social observation with more than 400 individual characters, chronicled the prosperity and decline of the (fictional) aristocratic Chia family. The epic story mirrored the first author's own experience and perceptions. Brought up in an aristocratic environment, he had born witness to the corruption and turmoil in society, and was poverty-stricken in later life. Much of his grief came from the death of his only son, and he himself died at about 50 years of age. The story boldly uncovered the power, greed and corruption of the nobles and the fall of morality and spirituality, and provided a voice for the suppressed, the pure and the honourable people. The diverse canvas of the story covered Chinese medicine, ceremony, religion, philosophy, foods and customs, providing valuable reference information for later generations.

James Legge 理雅各 (1815–1897 CE) – An outstanding sinologist of Scottish birth, James Legge was initially sent to China as a missionary. He soon came to be in charge of the Anglo-Chinese College in Malacca, which later moved to Hong Kong where he lived for some 30 years. Legge was the first Professor of Chinese at Oxford University (1876–1897). Legge's contributions to Chinese studies included his translation of the Chinese classics, notably the monumental book series *Sacred Books of the East*, published in 50 volumes between 1879 and 1891.

Dr Sun Yat-sen 孫中山 / 孫逸仙 (1866–1925 CE) – A national hero and revered as the 'Father of modern China' both in the People's Republic of China and in Taiwan, Sun Yat-sen was born in the Pearl River Delta in Kwangtung (later called Guangdong) province, on China's southern coast. He graduated from the Hong Kong College of Medicine for Chinese. Dr Sun's father, Dacheng, lived in Macau, which was to serve as Dr Sun's starting point to the West. During his years of education in Honolulu he learnt about Western democratic ideals, which greatly influenced him. Back to Macau, he was invited by the Kiang Wu Hospital to establish a Western Medicine Department, and became the first Chinese doctor to practice Western medicine in Macau. Later, he turned to political reform; 'the good of the people' was the basis for his revolutionary ideals. He overthrew the Qing Dynasty in 1911 and founded the Republic of China in 1912. Sun was the First President of the Republic of China and put an end to the 4000 years of imperial rule in China. He dedicated all his forty years of public life for the people. His vision of ideal government was nationalism, democracy, and socialism – the three principles 'of the people, by the people, and for the people'.

Lin Yutang 林語堂 (1895–1976 CE) – Committed to introducing Chinese classical literature and culture to the West, Lin Yutang was a philosopher, historian, novelist and prolific writer of more than 35 books in English and Chinese. He studied at St John's University (Shanghai) and Harvard University (USA), and obtained his PhD in Chinese studies at the University of Leipzig (Germany). He was a Professor of English literature at the University of Beijing from 1923–1926. After 1928 he lived mainly in the USA. His thinking was influenced by the landscape, especially mountains which made him feel 'humble', and by Taoism and Confucianism. With his book *My Country and My People* 吾國吾民 (1935), Lin Yutang became the first Chinese author to top the New York *Times* bestseller list. His other well-known books included *The Importance of Living* 生活的藝術 (1937), also a best-seller.

Fung Yu-lan 馮友蘭 (1895–1990 CE) – An eminent Chinese philosopher of the twentieth century, Fung Yu-lan was educated in Peking, obtained his PhD at Columbia University and, in 1928, became Professor of Philosophy at Tsinghua University in Peking. In 1946 Fung went to the USA to take up a post as Visiting Professor at the University of Pennsylvania. He spent the year 1948–49 as Visiting Professor at the University of Hawaii. His reputation was established by his two-volume *History of Chinese Philosophy* (1934), in which he used Western historical methods. Fung's book took certain metaphysical notions and a Taoist perspective. He also developed an account of the nature of morality and of the structure of human moral development.

Qian Mu 钱穆 (1895–1990 CE) – From a well-educated family, Qian Mu studied Chinese classics from his youth and later established himself as a high authority on Chinese history and culture. He was one of the founding members, together with Tang Chun-I (see below), of New Asia College in Hong Kong. Not long before New Asia College was integrated into the Chinese University (in 1963), Qian withdrew and later settled in Taiwan. Qian emphasised tradition and the past; for him, the characteristics of traditional Chinese culture resided in the 'heart', referring to the ordinary human heart. He valued inner virtue and self-cultivation as the origin for all actions on earth. His monumental works included *Culture and Education, The Twelve Chapters on Culture, Race and Culture* and *The Historical View of Chinese Culture* (all in Chinese).

Joseph Needham (1900–1995 CE) – A well-known scholar and scientist who came to have a 50-year association with China, Joseph Needham was sent by the British Council to war-torn China in 1943. He travelled widely, learnt about life in China, and established strong links with many distinguished Chinese scholars. He contributed to the first seven volumes of *The Science and Civilisation of China*; the last volume was unfinished but it is believed Dr Needham was still working on it the day before his death, at the age of 95, in his residence at the University of Cambridge.

Tang Chun-I 唐君毅 (1909–1978 CE) – A distinguished Professor in modern philosophy, Tang Chun-I's views are described as the 'second generation' of New Confucianism. (First generation Confucianism had more affinity with socialism, while second generation Confucianism tends towards liberalism and independence.) Tang Chun-I, with Qian Mu, established The New Asia College in Hong Kong in 1949 (later incorporated into the Chinese University). As a dedicated Confucian scholar, Tang emphasised 'human heart' as the essence of Chinese culture, together with emotion and action, and identified benevolence and humility as the ultimate sources of social reality. His writings, including his books *The Spiritual Value of Chinese Culture, The Development of Humanism* and *The Experience of Life* (all in Chinese), covered diverse Chinese cultural concepts and other topics.

Chinese Metaphors and Sayings

These metaphors and sayings were used by the Chinese people contributing to the studies reported in this book.

'A frog watching the sky in a well' 井底之蛙 – From an ancient Chinese story about a frog living in a well, who boasted it knew everything about the world based on what it could see looking up from the well. The message is to be humble and not to make assumptions without seeking enough information to establish the real situation.

'An emperor's life' 皇帝式的生活 – Describes a person who has a luxurious life, enjoying all the material comforts on earth and to whom everything is given. This implies a sense of superiority and good fortune.

'Body on the chopping board' 肉隨砧板上 – Implies a power relationship between, for instance, doctors and patients in which patients are relatively powerless, do not have much say, and have to listen to the doctors.

'Cheap bones' 賤人賤骨頭 – Refers to an unworthy or poor person with no social status, such that even their bones are considered worthless.

'Chicken at five' 五更雞 – Bird's nest soup (Traditional Chinese Medicine), prepared in a traditional manner with chicken and made ready for consumption at five in the morning, at which time of day it is believed to be beneficial to the body.

'Chinese east melon and tofu' 東瓜豆腐 – Conveys the image of bodily weakness in a female resulting from insufficient nourishment when young. Chinese east melon is solid on the outside but empty inside, and tofu is spongy; both food images imply a lack of internal substance. In other contexts, the metaphor can be used for misfortune or death.

'Darker than a ghost' 黑過鬼 – Depicts the complicated business world as a dark and surreal world like a 'ghost', where one could easily get lost in the darkness.

'Dead father and dead mother, and no family education' 死老豆死老母親沒家教 – A coarse and insulting expression of contempt towards another person. Parents are responsible for educating their children, so when a person acts socially unacceptably, it reflects poorly on his or her parents and upbringing. In terms of this insult, it appears the parents did their job so poorly they were as good as dead.

'Dress up like peacocks' 打扮成孔雀一樣 – People who dress colourfully, who almost appear to like showing off.

'Do not give enough rice to women before they turn eighty' 女人未到八十歲 不要給她吃太飽 – An old saying designed to belittle and control women, implying that a woman who is allowed to eat until she is full would not do her work properly.

'False little boy' 假小子 – Means a little girl who gives the appearance of being a boy; a metaphor connected with people's social experiences, commonly used in Shanghai, Mainland China.

'Gallbladder should be big and heart should be small 膽大心小 in action' – Undertaking work with courage to take up a challenge as well as with meticulous attention to detail in order to maintain balance. A 'big gallbladder' is equated with great courage, while a 'small heart' refers to the importance of meticulous and careful action.

'Heaven falls down like being covered by a blanket' 天跌下來像毯蓋 – How people can, in times of disaster, remain calm in mind and attitude, one's inner virtue unaffected by the external influences.

'Hundred patience turns into gold' 百忍成金 – Refers to 'patience' as a virtue and as a basis for harmonious social relationships; if one endures, one can expect to see good results. This 'patience' was emphasised in the traditional Chinese family system, which provided a training school for mutual tolerance.

'I did not know how high the sky was and how deep the earth was' 不知天有多高地有多深 – A proverb indicating ignorance, short-sightedness and lack of understanding, and perhaps someone who has been too protected and who has not thought fully about the complexities of life.

'Illness comes from the mouth' 病從口入 – Highlights the importance of foods in health. If we do not eat well, with the right balance of foods, illness may result. This saying also implies the importance of taking care of the inside (body) and the outside (external environments) at the same time.

'Lifetime rice ticket' 長期米票 – Finding a husband who will provide for a woman so that she won't need to work hard herself.

'Like a man at war' 像一個男人入戰場 – Compares the business world with a war, conjuring up images of danger, fighting and cruelty.

'One who puts in one's whole heart (with utmost effort) knows human nature' 盡其心者，知其性也 – A saying from Mencius, it is the heart that guides the self. The heart is not limited to directing the self alone but extends outside, embracing family, country and the world, touching on virtually all one's life. This high ideal of openness and unselfishness is a fine example of 'benevolence' in Confucianism.

'One with the strength of iron and yet soft inside' 鐵漢柔腸 – Describes a person who has great physical strength as well as a good and soft heart.

'Our best condition' 止於至善 – The full sentence from *The Great Learning* (chapter 1, attributed to Confucius) is: 'The principle of learning is to glorify and to develop our true moral nature, to effect good change, and to arrive at our very best condition'. According to the *Analects* (chapter 4), 'our best condition' can be realised when 'benevolence by the leaders, respect by the juniors, filial piety by children, kindness by parents, and trust between countries' is practised.

'Peaceful heart and harmonious *qi*' 心平氣和 – Has a social meaning regarding emotional health, and describes how acquiring a tranquil state will ensure peace in a family from the smooth flow of *qi* (一團和氣), for the social wellbeing of the family's members.

'People with eyebrows and eyes of a thief' 賊眉賊眼 – What is inside a person will show on the outside; good dress cannot disguise bad looks (or a bad heart).

'Single *yang* cannot not survive and lonely *yin* cannot grow' 獨陽不生，孤陰不長 – Refers to the co-existence and balance aspects of *yin* and *yang*. In ancient times it was believed that there would always be balance in the genders around practising Taoists – i.e. that wherever a male Taoist hermit was living in the mountains, there would be a female living somewhere nearby (related by one of the participants, a practitioner of Traditional Chinese Medicine).

'Teaching followers the full knowledge would end up with no masters' 教識徒弟沒師父 – Conveys reservations about teaching: firstly, implying that students with full knowledge would have an ungrateful attitude and would not defer to their teachers; and secondly, reflecting the inner insecurity of teachers and mistrust between teachers and students.

'The body is a storehouse' 身體像儲廢房 – Implies that for the body to function well, careful attention should be paid to avoiding 'surplus goods' or excess so that the storehouse is not overburdened and balance is maintained.

'The mountain becomes a treasure 滿山是寶; otherwise the whole mountain turns into grass 滿山是草 – Emphasises the importance of putting our knowledge into practice. Knowledge in action can turn something ordinary into something precious. Knowledge without action is wasteful.

'Three hearts and two attentions' 三心二意 – Three hearts means a loving heart, a consistent heart, and a determined heart; used by a participant in this book to refer to strategies for dealing with children with care, consistency and firmness. In other contexts, this metaphor refers to people, confused by too many options, being unable to make up their minds.

'To be a proper person' 做一個真正的人 – Means trying one's best in this world, from the words of the ancient Chinese scholar Luk Cheung Shan (陸象山) who said, 'Even if I don't know a word, I have to be a proper person'.

'Twenty-four examples of filial piety' 二十四孝 – Someone who shows complete filial piety is said to have acquired the 'twenty-four examples of filial piety'.

'Two captains at home' 一家有二個領袖 – 'Two captains' conveys a sense of two strong characters in one place and implies that they cannot live side by side because of the risk of disagreement.

'Universal love' 兼愛 – A doctrine of Mozi, the Chinese symbol 兼 shows a person holding two grains, which implies caring for others with a care that transcends time and space – endless, total care. Mozi's doctrine permitted no unfair treatment toward others, and promoted social behaviour that was caring, considerate, and equal.

'Using moral disciplines to improve human lives' 正德利用厚生 – From *Sheung Shu* (尚書), the oldest Chinese historical book (2300–1000 BCE), this concept implies one has to refine self first in order to help others; to be strict and to conquer self, and to be lenient toward others.

'Wind and rain' 風風雨雨 – Both metaphors for disaster and misfortune, especially related to an unstable social and political environment. A person who has gone through 'wind and rain' has experienced a turbulent life.

'Working like an ox' 做牛一樣 – Describes hardships and low social status in life. 'Ox' conjures the image of working hard and without complaint, a tough working life, and also of dehumanisation.

Glossary

Benevolence 仁 (or *yen* in Chinese) – is one of the highest ideals and practices in Confucianism and is considered the basis of all social interactions. The root of benevolence is filial piety toward parents, the respect of juniors toward seniors. Benevolence embodies many social meanings and is context specific. For Confucius, benevolence is realised through the practice of the cultivation of self, that is, to live is to realise benevolence. In Mencius's view, benevolence resides in the human heart and means endless compassion. Mozi's perspective differs in that benevolence is taken to mean all-embracing love that all people should enjoy equally and suffer equally.

'Cold' type 涼底 – belongs to *yin* constitutions. In order to balance the body, Traditional Chinese Medicine recommends a cold *yin* person should keep warm or 'hot', for which purpose *yang* foods (such as the animal meats of beef and lamb or spicy plants such as ginger and pepper) are recommended.

Dirty blood – relates to the toxic material that accumulates in our bodies as a result of bodily imbalance.

Dryness 燥 – a Traditional Chinese Medicine term, and believed to arise from excessive *yang*.

Equilibrium and harmony 中和 – according to *The Doctrine of the Mean*, various human emotions such as 'pleasure, anger, sorrow, or joy', if not expressed, are viewed as the state of 'Equilibrium'; if expressed in the proper manner without extremes, they are called 'Harmony'.

Filial piety 孝 – showing reverence to our parents. Filial piety is one of the key characteristics of Chinese culture, which has been referred to as 'the culture of filial piety'. The Chinese character for filial piety consists of two parts: the top part refers to 'the elderly', the lower part means 'son', illustrating that the son supports the elderly and the elderly is above the son. In the *Analects*, filial piety is defined as the utmost strength to treat parents with reverence. The extension of filial piety includes all elders, the living and the dead. Outside the family, filial piety is extended through benevolence to include the love of all mankind, the one big family ideal in Confucianism.

Gold–water 金水 – gold (or sometimes simply 'metal') and water refer to categories of quality and relationship in the five phases in Traditional Chinese Medicine: metal, water, wood, fire, and earth. Gold and water are considered mutually nourishing and promoting.

'Hot' type 熱底 – refers to a *yang* person and, following the philosophy of Traditional Chinese Medicine, foods of the opposite nature are recommended (lighter, cool *yin* foods such as fruit, vegetables, beans and eggs, which are easily digested and transformed into *qi* and blood) in order to preserve the body.

Harmonious energy 和氣 – is associated with social meanings of family and emotional health and beliefs. A popular Chinese saying is that harmonious energy generates wealth (和氣生財), which means that in a harmonious social relationship people will cooperate and work better to produce good outcomes.

Heat 熱 – according to Traditional Chinese Medicine theory, heat can be accumulated inside one's body. Excessive heat in the body is not necessarily synonymous with a high body temperature, and can be brought on by having too much *yang* food, causing imbalance in the body. See also 'pyretic *qi*'.

High liver fire 肝火上升 – in Traditional Chinese Medicine the liver is related to our emotional state and blood, and a disturbance to the liver may produce excess heat and cause bodily illness.

Human 人 – a key word in this book, as 'human centredness' is at the core of traditional Chinese culture. The conceptualisation of 'human' is complex and socially defined. In relation to self, 'human' means trying one's best in this world with strength that comes from 'self' and not from others, thus self-cultivation is critical. 'Human' is closely connected with 'benevolence', as reflected through filial piety within the family and in the social roles among family members. In a society, 'human' interaction requires consideration for others, mutual respect and harmonious intent. Therefore, the focus of 'human' is on the 'heart', linked to humanity and action.

Humanism 人道主義 – basically, consideration for others. Humanism is associated with the practice of 'benevolence', the love of life, the non-dualistic belief that all things on earth are of equal standing, the commitment to co-existence and accepting differences. The hallmark of humanistic action, according to Confucianism, would be to sacrifice oneself for benevolence.

Kidney energy 腎精 – significant in Traditional Chinese Medicine because the 'jing' essence, or semen, is believed to be stored in the kidneys, linking kidney energy with male reproduction. Kidney jing determines the growth of young people, and is used for future reproductive function.

Lai-See 利事 – a red envelope with money inside, a sign of blessing from the givers, for example given during the Chinese New Year and on some special occasions. If given from a junior to a senior, it is a sign of respect.

Pyretic *qi* 熱氣 – refers to an excess of yang or too much heat in the body. In Traditional Chinese Medicine, it signifies fire and heat in the lungs and stomach, and a deficit of *yin*. Pyretic *qi* is manifested as dryness in the mouth, sore throat, skin allergy and constipation. Foods that contribute to 'pyretic *qi*' are said to belong to the deep-fried, roasted, and spicy groups. The remedy in Traditional Chinese Medicine is to take soups that contain *yin* ingredients to cool the body and counteract excess *yang*.

Qi 氣 or energy – a vital concept in Traditional Chinese Medicine, *qi* is defined as the binding force of life (including heaven, earth and humans). Imbalance in life or an emptiness of *qi* reduces the body's ability to defend itself; the flow of *qi* can be blocked, and thus illness may result. Food believed to be a source of *qi*, and Traditional Chinese Medicine is considered food. The Chinese character is made up of two parts, the top part indicating 'rising vapour' and the lower part meaning 'rice', so that *qi* literally means 'vapour rising from rice'.

Resting month 坐月 – a month of rest and recuperation for the mother following childbirth in order to restore the energy of the body and to prevent disease. People believe that an inadequate 'resting month' will set the stage for poor health.

Social cement – refers to the human dimension of uniting people through affection, social support and symbols of human cohesion and, most often, by social action.

Three Lasting Establishments 三德 – 'to establish virtues, to establish contributions, and to establish knowledge' (立德, 立功, 立言), as mentioned in *Zuo Zhuan* (左傳), the earliest Chinese work of narrative history covering 722–468 BCE, these were guiding principles for life: to refine self and to contribute to others and society, including by giving helpful advice and sharing knowledge.

Wind 風 – commonly believed in Traditional Chinese Medicine to create disharmony in the body, and recorded in the *Historical Record* (史記) (around 100 BCE) compiled by Sze-ma Tsien (司馬遷) as a causative factor for illness. In Traditional Chinese Medicine, wind is considered capable of penetrating the body's surface and assisting the entry of other adverse forces, namely dampness, dryness, cold and heat.

Wuwei 無為 (or non-action) – in Tao, means doing things according to nature and harmonious relationships (i.e. actively rather than passively). *Wuwei* implies reflection and awareness, and good leaders having trust in people and allowing more freedom and space. The negative aspect is to not take action as a form of escapism or as a silent protest against reality.

Yang **energy** 陽精力 – male energy and related energies; *yang* energy is the basis for vitality in boys and virility in adult males. According to *Nei Jing*, *yang* energy belongs to heavenly energy, which nourishes one's head, and to foods that provide *yang* energy such as animal meats.

Yin **and** *yang* 陰陽 – perceived to be the originators and principles of all things, '*yin* and *yang*' is a fundamental concept in Traditional Chinese Medicine, underlying how the phenomenon of life is thought to function in relation to the environment. Formulated as a conceptual framework in *I Ching* (*The Book of Changes*) and further developed in the first Chinese medical classic, *Nei Jing* (*Yellow Emperor's Canon of Internal Medicine*), *yin* and *yang* are described by symbolic lines in sixty-four six-line diagrams called 'hexagrams'. A solid line (—) represents *yang*, heaven (referring to strength, movement and the positive and bright side of all things). A broken line (– –) represents *yin*, the earth (representing receptiveness, quietness, darkness and gentleness). All changes in natural phenomena operate in the ceaseless motion and complementarity of *yin* and *yang*, like heaven and earth, sun and moon. Once *yin* and *yang* are out of balance, disease is inevitable.

Yin **energy** 陰精力 – female energy and related energies; in *Nei Jing*, *yin* energy belongs to earth and nourishes one's feet. In Traditional Chinese Medicine, *yin* energy is related to blood, and Traditional Chinese Medicine is sometimes used for nourishment and 'blood-building'.

Yuan 緣 – the intuitive feeling or luck that binds people together.

Index

211

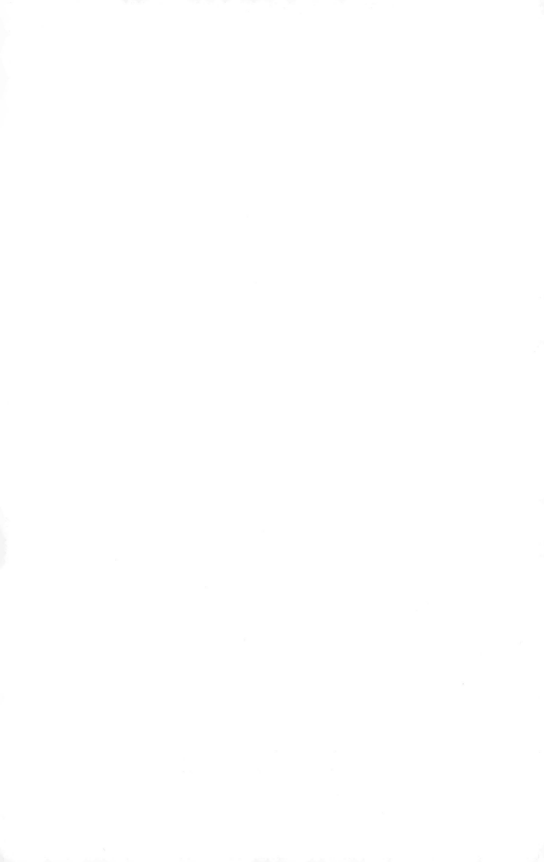

T - #0377 - 101024 - C228 - 229/152/12 - PB - 9780977574223 - Gloss Lamination